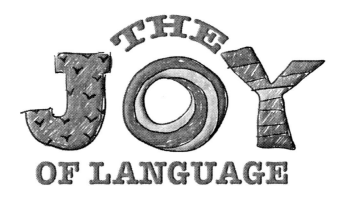

THE JOY
OF LANGUAGE

The Guide to Language and Learning
for Parents and Caregivers

Tara J. Tuck, CAGS, CCC-SLP

MArco River Press

The Joy of Language:
The Guide to Language and Learning
for Parents and Caregivers

Tara J. Tuck, CAGS, CCC-SLP

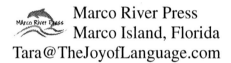 Marco River Press
Marco Island, Florida
Tara@TheJoyofLanguage.com

Cover design and interior layout: www.TheBookProducer.com
Printed in the United States of America

The Joy of Language: The Guide for Language and Learning
for Parents and Caregivers / Tara J. Tuck

ISBN 978-0-9969620-0-1 (paper)
ISBN 978-0-9969620-1-8 (retail e-book)

1. Parenting 2. Family and Relationships 3. Child Development 4. Child Rearing 5. Language Development 6. Speech 7. Speech Disorders 8. Language Disorders 9. Education 10. Learning 11. Reading

DEDICATION

To my husband Bill,
the love of my life.
This was all so worth the wait.

ACKNOWLEDGEMENTS

Annie Sullivan – My first reader and editor, and my cherished friend, who is constantly creating, delighting and discovering peace, joy and beauty – and sharing it every day.

Pat Steuert – For your valuable comments and encouragement, and for your friendship.

My husband Bill – For your love and understanding, for always being there to help and advise me, for seeing me through all challenges, and for your constant belief in me.

The many children I have worked with throughout the years and their parents, who have trusted me and partnered with me. Together we have seen and celebrated the development of countless successful communicators and learners.

Thank you.

CONTENTS

PART 1: Learning Language ~ 17

Chapter 1
The Basics: What EVERY Parent and Caregiver Needs to Know . . 19

Chapter 2
Articulation and Phoneme Development: Making Sounds, Syllables and Words

Chapter 3
Learning New Words (Vocabulary) and Meanings:
Semantic Development

Chapter 4
Using Sentences: Morphemes + Syntax = Grammar

PART 2: Learning With Language ~ 139

Chapter 8

Chapter 9

ILLUSTRATIONS

INTRODUCING
The Joy of Language

Meet the Author

Tara Tuck began her career as an educator teaching elementary school in Massachusetts. She earned a bachelor's degree at Lesley College, a master's degree in Speech and Language Pathology from Boston University and a Certificate of Advanced Graduate Studies in Administration, Planning and Social Policy from the Harvard Graduate School of Education. Ms. Tuck developed and taught one of the first self-contained classes for students with severe language disabilities, and worked for many years as a speech-language pathologist specializing in classroom inclusion, becoming a district inclusion specialist in Florida. She has extensive experience with all ages of children, from toddlers through high school and has developed and taught numerous workshops for teachers on language and literacy skills. Ms. Tuck currently teaches graduate courses in Linguistics and English as a Second Language for Lesley University in addition to her work with parents, caregivers and teachers through *The Joy of Language* publications, seminars and web site.

In the Author's Own Words: Why I Am Committed to *The Joy of Language*

While working with and speaking with so many parents over the years, I realized that they rarely find a book or program that answers the myriad of questions they have about the development of speech, language and learning. There are some excellent books focusing on language development, but so many seem to be either written as college textbooks or are not easily used as reference books for parents and caregivers. This book was written for you. Since parents have so many questions and concerns about how their children are developing the capacity to learn and to communicate, this information needs to be easily accessible. *The Joy of Language* will help you to find answers quickly and to put the information into practice immediately – while having **FUN** with your child.

Not only is this guide user friendly, but you can also **rely on** the information in this book. Parents, caregivers and teachers need to be aware of the validity of the developmental strategies suggested by books, materials, kits, web sites and programs that claim to help children to become smarter, to read earlier, or to excel in countless ways. It is always important for parents and caregivers to make sure the books and programs they are using to help their children develop linguistically, cognitively, physically and emotionally are well researched and are, in fact, providing sound practices for child development. You can be sure that the information used in the writing of this book is from well documented research articles in peer reviewed journals and professional publications, as well as from the author's personal experience of many years in the field of language development. It is important to me, and it should be to you, that the information and strategies in this book can be **trusted**.

Doesn't the teaching of speech and language come naturally to most parents?

Much of it does. But really being knowledgeable about how children learn language allows an adult to focus on specific ways to encourage language at different ages, and also to keep track of each important stage of language acquisition. In fact, some studies have found mothers not to be the best judge of childhood language. But as a parent who is using this guide to ensure optimum language development, you are already on your way to providing the best for your child. As you would expect, better parenting sets the foundation for success of early childhood education and later success in school. This foundation then will support your child's ability to construct meaning through oral and written language. Generally, good oral language skills before first grade = good reading skills thereafter. Even children who attend preschool spend most of their time in the home environment. For that reason, parents need to understand how crucial the home environment is for their child's success. Do not leave this crucial period (birth to five) of your child's language development up to teachers. Your child needs you: your expertise, your modeling, your encouragement and your love.

Is *The Joy of Language* mostly for parents?

This book (and the accompanying website, www.TheJoyof Language.com), is a wonderful resource for parents. It should be used as a reference throughout the first years of a child's life. It is my hope, however, that any caregivers of babies and young children (nannies, babysitters, preschool teachers, pediatricians, and many others) will also use this information for providing the best care for children and for consulting with parents. And parents who have their child in the care of others for a good part of the day or evening should share this information. Speech and language development is a 24-hour a day process, and parents need to know that whoever is caring for their children is doing all the right things to encourage that development. All parties also need to be aware of whether the child is reaching important milestones, or if an early intervention specialist should be contacted, not necessarily to provide therapy, but to demonstrate how best to identify daily routines as contexts for learning language.

Will I be able to find answers quickly in this book?

Yes. This book is organized in a way that makes finding the answers simple. It begins with the basics: how babies' brains develop, what language actually is (explaining all features of speech and language), and detailed developmental charts. It is a user friendly guide for parents and caregivers who are supporting and encouraging excellent language and learning skills in children from birth to school age. Each chapter, including this introduction, is organized by questions parents might ask about speech or language, and the Table of Contents includes those questions so information can be found easily. Many of the questions, in fact, will spark an interest so the reader will immediately turn to that page for instant discovery. Also note that answers to questions are written with both male and female pronouns (he, she, him, her) to make it easier to read – using "he/she" throughout the book would make it cumbersome. Naturally, all information pertains to both boys and girls unless otherwise specified.

At the end of most chapters are activities that accelerate the learning of that aspect of language and that are enjoyable for both children and caregivers. These sections are under the heading of **Sharing the Joy**. Some of the Sharing the Joy activities will be repeated in other chapters because the same activities can, and should, be used to encourage different aspects of language. For example, giving simple directions ("Give the cup to Daddy.") can be used to stimulate listening and attention, sentence structure, vocabulary, or even articulation of the sounds /g/ and /k/. It is important to understand that everyday activities and ways of communicating can encourage the development of many language skills, and that just the right emphasis can address what your child needs at that moment. It will also become clear to you that **Sharing the Joy** with your baby, toddler or preschooler does not require expensive toys or programs!

Is *The Joy of Language* a "basic" guide, or does it also contain more in-depth information?

It is really both. There are medical and linguistic terms throughout, but they will be defined and used in a way that will make them easy to understand. Knowing these terms will also help you to communicate more effectively with speech-language pathologists, teachers, pediatricians, psychologists and other child development specialists if the need arises. Much of the vocabulary in this book is also defined in the Glossary, so there are many opportunities for learning and reviewing concepts. Understanding the vocabulary means understanding the concepts and processes related to speech, language and learning. As you will see, *The Joy of Language* includes information necessary for parents to feel comfortable participating in IEP (Individualized Education Program) and assessment meetings in school settings. Parents need to be experts in child development in order to partner with professionals and to ensure the best for their children.

Are there other resources I can use as I read this book?

Absolutely. For a wealth of additional information about speech, language and learning, please visit the web site www.TheJoyofLanguage.com. There you will find a very informative blog, answers to parents' questions, charts, informal assessments, additional resources for parents, and much more.

And please, please share this book and the ideas from it with your child's older siblings, relatives and caregivers. Whoever comprises your "village" is going to affect your child's communication skills, so it is up to you to spread the word about how to be teachers, models and cheer leaders. Share the book, share the knowledge, be a role model, and be amazed by what your child is learning every day. Share the Joy!

Tara Tuck, CAGS, CCC-SLP

PART 1:
Learning Language

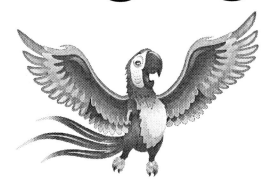

CHAPTER 1

The Basics:
What EVERY Parent and
Caregiver Needs to Know

Babies are born ready to learn language. We just need to set the stage for them to flourish by providing them with an environment of caring, physical and mental stimulation, and models of communication. When babies feel safe and cared for, they want to communicate with their caregivers. When they experience love, they take the chances needed to practice language. When they hear and see others interacting with them, they work hard at figuring out how to do the same.

How can I set a secure foundation for my baby?

Language develops best in an emotionally safe environment. During the first two years of a child's life, while language is beginning to develop, the social and emotional needs of the child are crucial. Survival is based on emotional connection – knowing that he or she is safe and everything is okay. Then language development can flourish. When we think they are so cute (Awwww!) babies are actually exhibiting some very skillful acts of self-preservation. They are born with the natural ability to alleviate fear and anxiety by bonding with others. Babies thrive on this connection with family, family friends, caregivers, and animals.

Early experiences shape the brain's expectations and "architecture" by building crucial pathways. Babies are born curious, motivated to learn, initiating communication, imitating, and interacting. When babies delight in interaction, they become more skillful at it. But when babies are not nurtured, or when they are not made to feel safe and loved, their brains become structured to expect danger; they are ready for defense. These babies will be anxious, trusting and exploring the world less. So these early experiences form the emotional base for the development of both language and intellect.

Once a baby is secure in expecting that his needs will be met, he can begin to look for novel experiences through curiosity. As long as his caregiver responds to his needs in a timely manner – reading cues accurately and providing what is appropriate – the stage is set. Of course, your baby also needs to know that everything can't be predicted; many things are spontaneous. But flexibility is only possible after a foundation of safety is established.

Once your baby can crawl and become more active, she will need security provided in a different way. She will explore, but will keep looking back at you to make sure you're there and that you will acknowledge her. She is learning how to separate while still staying connected.

During this stage, your baby will also learn, from reactions of caregivers, what is socially acceptable behavior. Then, as a toddler, your child will need the safety of guided self-regulation with consistent involvement of her caregivers. She will learn that you can't scribble all over another child's paper or grab someone's toy away from them. There are more socially appropriate ways to interact, and they involve using words. These are rules of her culture, her society and her family. She needs to learn that while her own needs are being respected, she also must respect the needs of others. This ability to regulate one's own behavior and to practice constraint is called "executive function." This will be discussed in more detail in chapter 6.

When will my baby begin to learn language?

Even before birth! Your baby can hear your voice and other environmental sounds in utero. He will not be able to see well at birth, but he will be able to hear everything, and even to discriminate one sound from another. We can see newborns tuning in to human communication. They seem to seek human faces, especially when we are talking to them.

Babies' brains are truly incredible. At birth they actually contain more neurons than they need, and a "pruning" process takes place within the first two years. Because of baby's experiences during this time, including the language she hears, the neurons needed to remember and use these bits of information are retained, and other neurons become dormant. Your baby's experiences will actually shape her brain, and you can provide just the right experiences for your baby to thrive cognitively, linguistically, physically and emotionally.

By six months your baby will even begin to recognize, and tune in to, the language, or languages, of his environment. The baby hears people speaking and he turns toward the source of the sounds. If a person is speaking directly to the baby, making facial expressions, and exaggerating intonations and gestures, the baby is interested and wants to figure out what it all means. The baby's brain is ready, willing and able to learn this remarkable skill – the miracle of human language!

Babies prefer to listen to infant-directed speech (discussed further in Chapters 3 and 4), the sing-songy speech that we use when talking to babies. They begin to attend to language by hearing "the big picture," the whole, the *gestalt* – not yet understanding individual words. To a baby this is just a series of sounds, but every once in a while it will contain a very familiar word that she has heard often, like *Mommy*, *Daddy* or the baby's name. ("Does Sally want some more juice?") Baby listens, and soon baby talks.

So how can you know when your baby is beginning to understand language? Each child learns language at his own speed, but there are developmental norms that we use to note milestones. You should note your child's progress, but remember that there is a range of normal development. For instance, girls tend to develop language slightly earlier than boys, probably because of earlier specialization of brain cells. Boys soon catch up, though. The oldest child also generally develops language earlier than later born children, probably because parents have more time to devote to him, interacting one-on-one. Twins often display somewhat delayed language skills because they interact with each other so frequently, and they keep each other occupied and communicating in a variety of ways. So there are a number of factors that affect the speed of language development, but babies throughout the world learn the language of their family and culture in the same way. Parents and caregivers around the planet are experiencing the same miracle of language development.

Why do I need this much information about how speech and language develop?

Because when we really understand something we can use it wisely and easily, and become an expert at it. It will also become a lot more enjoyable sharing language with your baby when you understand how important it is. You will be motivated to continue working on it every chance you get. In a way, it's like the difference between being able to cook vs. being a great chef. If you can read a recipe, you can cook; if you understand ingredients, combinations of tastes, texture and colors, and know how to make dining fun and exciting, you can be a chef! You don't want to be able to just cook up some ways to help develop your child's communication skills; you want to be the expert who is creating a masterpiece! Your child deserves the best – and the best is YOU.

Many parents, even parents who have had more than one child, don't really know what children's language is supposed to sound like. Parents have many questions about speech and language: "Should I be able to understand everything my 4-year-old is saying?" "Why does he keep saying, 'Him go to the store'?" "I think my toddler just hears what she wants to hear." "Is there anything wrong with calling water 'wawa'?"

Some parents don't think it's a good idea to compare their children with others, and other parents are constantly comparing children. The best way to determine whether your child is on the right track is by really understanding each stage of speech and language development, and by watching, listening, talking and playing with your child every day as you observe this miracle.

Is speech the same as language?

No, although speech is an integral part of language, and the words are sometimes used interchangeably – even in some chapters of this book. You will understand the meaning of the words from the context, however. *Speech* usually refers to the pronunciation of words (articulation), the easy flow of speech (fluency vs. stuttering), and the quality of the sound of one's voice (normal sounding vs. hoarse, harsh, or unusual in pitch or volume). Speaking requires us to translate our thoughts into sound sequences that are understood by others.

Then what is language?

I'm sure you know that language has to do with talking, but it is much more than that. It is the brain's ability to understand and express oral and written symbols, words, and sentences, and to do so appropriately in a variety of contexts. Language is speaking, listening, understanding, thinking, reading and writing. It is essentially most of what makes us human, gives us the ability to interact with each other, enables us to learn whatever we think is important and to achieve our goals and dreams.

Language is our phonological system (sounds in words), our grammar and sentence formulation in both speaking and writing, our vocabulary, the organization of our thoughts, and our own monitoring of all of this. Using language is a very complicated process, but most of us just take it for granted. We learn to speak, read and write, and, unless we have a language or learning problem, we don't think about it much until we try to learn a new language.

It is difficult for most of us even to imagine the complexities of language, and children learn this enormously intricate system largely without any instruction at all. That doesn't mean we don't have to help it along. Doing everything you can to develop your child's language from birth, through infancy, into toddlerhood and beyond is a priceless gift you will be giving to your child. Give it with joy! But you aren't really "teaching" your child language skills, you are providing him with a perfect environment for learning. It is much too complicated a system for us ever to be able to teach, as you will come to understand while reading this book. No one "taught" you to speak. They couldn't have. So how did you learn – and what did you learn? What is happening in our brains as we are communicating thoughts?

First let's look at what language really is.

Language Is ...

- **Phonemes** – the sounds of any language
- **Morphemes** – meaningful parts of words

- **Syntax** – sentence formulation and word order
- **Semantics** – vocabulary, ideas and meaning
- **Pragmatics** – the social use, purpose or intent of language

These five aspects can be demonstrated by this diagram which illustrates how we can easily remember exactly what language *is*.

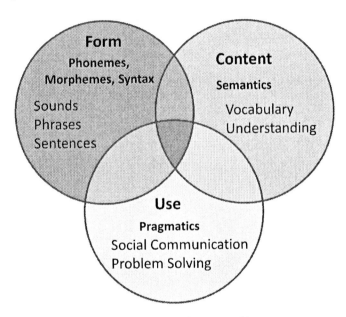

**Figure 1: Form – Content – Use
Diagram of Major Aspects of Language**

- **Form** – Phonemes, Morphemes and Syntax (What speech and language sounds like and also looks like on paper)
- **Content** – Semantics (vocabulary, meaning of what is said and written)
- **Use** – Pragmatics (saying or writing the right thing at the right time)

You can see that all sections of the diagram overlap. That is because it is difficult to separate one from another: the **reason** we speak (Use) is expressed by **what** we are saying (Content) and **how** we are saying it (Form). Labeling and defining each aspect of language, however, helps us to understand the process and what we need to know in order to effectively communicate.

We also develop the ability to **think about** language; we have an **awareness** of language. This is called **metalinguistic awareness**. Metalinguistic awareness is the awareness that language is an object that can be used and manipulated. The prefix *meta* means beyond, like looking at something from beyond, or outside of it. Very young children have very limited metalinguistic awareness, but it is one of the most important aspects of the development of language for reading and writing. It is one of our cognitive abilities that begins to develop around age four. You can have a conversation with a 3-year-old, but she will most likely not be able to tell you which sounds are in her words or to count the number of words in her sentences. She may even be able to fill in a rhyming word at the end of a children's poem, but she is unlikely to be able to tell you how she did it. She can use language, but not talk about it. She doesn't have the metalinguistic awareness to do that.

How will I know that my child has developed metalinguistic awareness?

By the time a child begins kindergarten, he should have enough metalinguistic awareness to be able to use some letters as beginning sounds of words, to understand that words are made up of continuous streams of sounds, and to think of some words that rhyme with "cat" or "mouse." The processes of reading and writing will enhance his ability to think about his use of language, as will participation in group work, oral presentations, plays, Readers Theater, etc. By the time he is in seventh grade and "learning grammar," he is actually just labeling what he already knows. He is not really learning grammar; he is learning new ways to talk about grammar. He is giving names to it, analyzing and synthesizing parts, manipulating words and structures, building on concepts, and learning to write for a specific audience – applying his metalinguistic knowledge.

Why do I have to know all of these terms?

Even though this is new vocabulary for most people, it is helpful to know the terms in order to really understand what language is all about, to look up further information on your own, and to possibly communicate with speech-language pathologists (speech therapists), pediatricians, or other child development specialists if the need should arise. You probably won't have to be a part of an IEP (Individual Education Plan) team at your child's school – but you might. If this should happen, you will be very happy that you understand the jargon and can wisely contribute to the development of a plan of education for your child. Don't worry. You will quickly get used to the vocabulary and it will become second nature to you. This is an expansion of your *semantic* knowledge. See? You are already on your way to becoming an expert!

Will I need the right games, books, toys and other tools to make sure my child's brain develops well?

No! What your child's brain needs, in addition to health and nutrition, is a loving, caring environment in which she can move, explore, communicate, listen, interact, sing, talk and play. Your child needs stimulating experiences with her five senses, and these experiences can be found essentially everywhere – with no special equipment or expensive toys or programs. In fact, even if you wanted to, you couldn't buy any program to teach language to your baby; but you can, and will, be an extraordinary *facilitator* of language – you and your baby joyfully getting to know each other!

How does this all happen?

Essentially, the brain is a pattern-detecting device. Babies listen to the patterns of language, and their brains organize these patterns into "rules" of the language or languages they hear. So we must provide the perfect circumstances for our baby's brain to detect the patterns she hears when her family and caregivers are talking. We emphasize certain words, we sometimes speak slowly, and we repeat sounds, words and phrases. We do whatever we can to allow the child's brain to figure out the patterns that will become her speech and language.

A child's brain is primed and ready to detect the patterns and to acquire language, but there is also a critical period for doing this: the first years of life, beginning at birth. The young brain *must* be exercised by interacting with the environment during these critical years. It must develop and use these brain connections or lose them. The baby's experiences will determine which connections will become well developed and which will not. When connections are made repeatedly, they become permanent. Language pathways will continue to be formed until the child is about ten years of age, but the most important developmental period is from birth to kindergarten. That's why it is so important not only to be a great facilitator, but also a great observer of your child's language development. It is up to you to make sure it is on target.

Because of your child's need to communicate, language is learned functionally. You have to learn to ride a bicycle by riding; you have to learn to swim by swimming; you have to learn to talk by talking. You can tell someone how to swim so that they can describe swimming to you and say that they now know how to swim. But they still may not be able to swim if they fall into deep water. Once they experience swimming, though, it is much easier to understand when others talk about how to swim. Language, like swimming, is functional and experiential.

It is also helpful for you to know the theories that are used to explain how language is learned. They may sound complicated, but they really are quite understandable. Although not one is sufficient by itself to explain how language develops, bits and pieces of each are factors in this miraculous process. As they are described below, really think about what each is describing. You will be encouraging your child's language development by using bits and pieces of each of them every day. You can also watch each theory at work as your baby learns to communicate with more and more precision.

Do we really know how and why we learn language?

Not exactly, but there are three main theories, ideas based on research and observation, about the conditions needed for language acquisition: **Behavioral Theory**, **Cognitive Theory** and **Innate Theory**.

Behavioral Theory, based on the work of B.F. Skinner, is the premise that an action of a human or animal will either be rewarded, not rewarded, or punished. If it is rewarded, it will continue (e.g., if you get a bonus at work for doing a great job, you will continue doing a great job). If it is not rewarded, it will eventually fade (e.g., if you do a great job and no one notices, you probably won't keep trying so hard). If it is punished, it will be extinguished (e.g., if, because you do your job so efficiently, your boss gives you twice as much work, you will stop being as efficient). So if a baby says, "Dada," and

Daddy smiles, picks up the baby and lifts him into the air, the baby will most likely say, "Dada" again to get a similar reaction. If when the baby says, "Dada" he receives no reaction from anyone, within a short time he will stop saying this. If when the baby says, "Dada" he is yelled at and told never to say that again (a very unlikely event, we hope), he is unlikely ever to say, "Dada" again.

Well, this theory seems quite plausible. But it isn't sufficient to explain how babies learn to speak. Why not? Isn't it true that when we reward them, they speak more? Yes, but when it comes to language, there are many exceptions to these behavioral rules. Let's think about that. We don't only do things because we are going to get something for doing them; we also do things because they are fun, challenging and interesting. Since intrinsic motivation is also such an important factor in human learning, it is certainly another factor in the development of language. We know that if a baby attempts to communicate and gets no reward for doing so, he will eventually stop trying. If he is rewarded for not communicating (e.g., if he gets attention from the family by siblings giving him things he points to) his language will most likely develop more slowly. But consider this: babies who are 18 months old are usually given what they want after naming it with only one word. But they still develop two- and three-word utterances, and eventually full grammatical sentences. **So what's going on?**

Maybe we need some ideas from the next theory to fill in the pieces. According to **Cognitive Theory**, based on the work of Jean Piaget (and the similar **Interactionist Theory** of Lev Vygotsky), the child develops language and problem-solving skills by interacting with his environment. The child hears language, sees people interacting with each other, and has many opportunities to communicate with others using words, gestures and facial expressions. He learns the names of things and how to categorize them (dogs that look very different from each other are still dogs); he names actions and emotions; he learns how to describe things; he learns as he interacts with other people. As he experiences consequences and cause and effect relationships he begins to think with language, to solve problems, and to predict what will happen next. The child learns, he learns language, and he learns through language – simultaneously. **More than anything else, he needs to have experiences in a language-rich environment.**

So we know that babies have to be rewarded, they have to have experiences, and they have to practice communicating. But really, what is it about a baby's brain that enables it to learn language? Well, let's look at the third theory, the **Innate Theory**, based on the research of Noam Chomsky. This theory proposes that because we are human, we are born with the ability to learn human language and with the strong desire to use it. Infants' brains are prepared to listen, to label, to interpret, and to develop grammar, as well as to develop a tremendous vocabulary to express their thoughts, needs and emotions. The ability to pick individual words out of phrases and sentences spoken by people around him, to use those words, and then to expand those single words into phrases is an unimaginably complex, even miraculous process that all normally developing babies experience. We speak because we were born human. Yes, we are truly remarkable!

Do I have to know about my baby's brain in order to make sure he develops good language skills?

This could have been a program of recipes about what parents and caregivers should be doing to help develop children's language skills. Web sites for parents, books about child development, and blogs from pediatricians are plentiful, and many of them contain very important and useful information about how to be a great parent or caregiver.

Knowing about the brain and about how we acquire language, however, will provide you with so many more resources, skills and flexibility for ensuring that both you and your child find the JOY of language and learning for a lifetime. This information will also start you thinking about your own brain – a process of self-discovery that will help you to help your child on an even deeper level. You won't only know *what* to do, but *why*. And if something doesn't seem to be appealing or working at that moment, you will quickly be able to devise another way to help your child acquire the vocabulary, use better sentence structure, listen more carefully, or say the right thing.

You'll come to realize that language is truly fascinating. Brains are fascinating. Human potential is fascinating. Individual differences are fascinating. Your baby, your toddler, your child – and YOU – are fascinating.

What parts of the brain are used for language?

Well, let's look at an overview of our brains.

A child's brain is quite different from an adult's brain. It is continually growing and developing, and it has about twice as many synapses (connections) as an adult. During the first year of life, the number of synapses double in order to be ready for the rapid creation of knowledge and skills. A baby's brain contains about 100 billion nerve cells, known as neurons, and each of them can connect with 15,000 other cells. A three-year-old's brain contains about 1,000 trillion connections! This creates an incredibly complex network – that is largely formed by experience. You might be tempted to skip over this section, but you'll find here some really interesting information about your baby's brain – and YOURS!

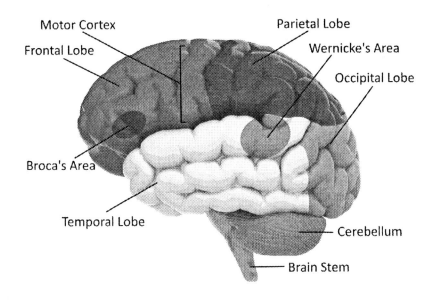

Figure 2: Left Hemisphere of Brain

The brain is comprised of three main parts: the **cerebrum**, or **cerebral cortex** (both left and right hemispheres), the **cerebellum,** and the **brain stem**. We will focus mainly on the **cerebral areas** of the brain for discussing language development because this is where our cells for language and cognition are located. We do not use the two lower areas of the brain for what we consider thinking and problem solving, although the **cerebellum** does contribute to the muscle coordination needed for the act of speaking. (It is largely responsible for balance, equilibrium and coordination of muscles for our daily activities.) The **brain stem** is instrumental in integrating information from our five senses. It also regulates functions that we don't have to think about controlling: breathing, digestion, heartbeat, blood pressure, swallowing, pupil size, and other basic bodily functions.

CEREBRUM

The **cerebrum** (also called the **cerebral cortex** or the **neocortex**), which is responsible for our cognitive functioning (thought, problem solving, language skills, action planning) comprises about 90 percent of brain tissue. It is separated into two halves, or **hemispheres**, and these hemispheres are connected by a dense group of nerve fibers called the **corpus callosum**. The **cerebrum** is also divided into four sections, or lobes: **frontal**, **parietal**, **temporal** and **occipital**. These lobes are in both the right and left hemisphere, but their function in each hemisphere is somewhat different from their function in the other. Most aspects of language are processed in the **left hemisphere**, but many of our perceptions that affect language are processed in the right hemisphere. This will be explained further in this chapter.

TEMPORAL LOBE

The two temporal lobes are located at just about ear level on both sides of the brain. They are responsible for hearing, taste, smell, receptive language (processing, understanding and thinking with language) and short-term memory. The right temporal lobe is mainly involved in visual memory, such as pictures or faces, while the left temporal lobe is mainly involved in verbal memory, such as words and names. It is the primary auditory cortex, which is responsible for the understanding of oral language, or semantic comprehension. (Semantics, the meaning of words and sentences, will be explained in chapter 3.)

WERNICKE'S AREA

Wernicke's Area is located at the top of the temporal lobe in the left hemisphere, between the temporal and parietal lobes. It is responsible for our recognition and understanding of language. It also allows us to monitor our own speech and language.

FRONTAL LOBE

The frontal lobe is responsible for intelligence, problem solving, decision making, monitoring behavior, attention, emotions, sympathy and empathy, movement and speech. It is responsible for a great amount of what we call "personality."

BROCA'S AREA

Broca's area is located in the lower portion of the left frontal lobe. Its function is to allow us to formulate sentences, which means using words in a grammatically correct order, and to sequence sounds. When we want to communicate thoughts and ideas, we don't only need the vocabulary, but we also need phrases and sentences in order to communicate entire, detailed messages. Broca's area allows us to formulate sentences and to sequence speech sounds into words.

MOTOR CORTEX

The motor cortex plans movements (motor planning) and signals the body to perform motor sequences. The sequences of movements of our articulators (lips, tongue and jaw, as well as other muscles of the mouth and throat) originate in this area of the brain and are carried to the spinal cord to activate our muscles.

PARIETAL LOBE

The two parietal lobes are located at the top of the brain, behind the frontal lobes. The parietal lobes have many functions: sensations like touch and pressure, spatial relationships, texture, weight, size and shape, taste, pain, and the feelings inside our muscles as they move. The part of the brain that lies partly in the left parietal and partly in the left temporal lobe enables us to analyzing words as we read, the way beginning readers try to "attack" words.

OCCIPITAL LOBE

The occipital lobe is the region in the back of the head which processes visual information. It is often called the visual cortex. This includes visual reception (knowing that one is seeing something), visual association (such as recognition of objects), and perception of shapes, colors and movement. A portion of the brain that lies partly in the left occipital and partly in the left temporal lobe allows skilled readers to identify words immediately. Written language will be discussed in chapter 8, and you might want to refer back to this section as you learn more about how your child will learn to read.

Which is the "language" hemisphere?

You've probably heard that language is a left hemisphere skill, but a very important part of language is processed in the right hemisphere. The left hemisphere processes formulas and rules, so it formulates sentences by using linguistic rules. It memorizes facts, algebraic formulas and sequences of steps in reading strategies. The *form* of language (phoneme sequences, morphemes and syntax) originates in the left hemisphere. The *content*, or meaning (semantics), of words also originates in the left hemisphere, but the right hemisphere must *choose* among a variety of words or meanings depending upon the verbal or written context, or the social situation – the pragmatics, or use, of language.

The right hemisphere helps us to understand things in context and to perceive the overall function and intention of the communication. It is as if the right hemisphere is always asking, "What did she really mean by that?" This is the *use* of language. Our interpretation of words and sentences depends on who is speaking, what the social situation is, the speaker's intonation and body language, which meaning of the word makes sense in the sentence, and many other factors. So the real, or underlying, meaning of spoken or written language is dependent upon the right hemisphere. This will be explained more fully in the Chapter 6, Social Language.

What should I be looking for during those critical years?

All children do not develop skills at the same rate, but there are guidelines for normal language development. Some children develop skills a little earlier, and some develop them a little later. The following chart should help you in determining whether your child is on target, and it will also help you to decide which skills to focus on in your interactions with him. Since physical, emotional and cognitive growth are all necessary for the development of language, these areas of skill are included in the chart. Remember that language development begins at birth, so everything you do with your baby is helping him to become a communicator.

STAGES OF LANGUAGE DEVELOPMENT

Birth to 3 months:

0 – 2 months gurgles, coos and makes "vegetative" sounds

Recognizes parents' voices

Recognizes parents' faces at 2 months

Smiles or is quieted when mother speaks

Has limited vision, so needs your face to be close to hers for her to see you (visual acuity of newborn is about 20/200)

Watches your eyes when your face is close to her face; interested in facial expressions

Follows an object moving slowly 6 inches from his face

Holds head up and pushes up when on tummy

Looks at his own hands

Brings things to mouth

Smiles at people

Smiles as you fuss about her

Discriminates between speech sounds, like /b/ and /p/

Cries differently for different reasons (happy, upset, bored, hungry, dirty diaper, in pain, etc.)

Decreases crying at about 2 months

Follows noise of a rattle at 2 months

Makes at least 2 different vowel-like sounds at 2 months

Reacts to loud noises with arm movements and facial expressions; looks toward the source at 3 months

Stays awake longer at 3 months

Starts to imitate facial expressions of adults near baby's face

Enjoys listening to music and your singing

Gets excited when favorite song is played

Learns to attend to your gaze, touch and tone of voice (as basis for conversation)

Starts to see color, first red and green

STAGES OF LANGUAGE DEVELOPMENT

3 to 6 months:

Looks toward sounds

Listens attentively to different noises

Smiles readily, crying decreases

Coos and gurgles when adult reads to her

Shares joint attention, focusing on what the adult points to
and talks about

Attends to tones of voice

Babbles and coos with speech sounds at 4 months, many
with multiple syllables

Pauses babbling when you reply, beginning "conversation"

Babbles when you leave a gap in speaking

Attends to sound toys and music by moving arms and legs

Laughs and chuckles in amusement

Screams when angry

Looks at himself in mirror with fascination

Pushes head and shoulders off ground when lying face down,
so notices and touches, or tries to reach, more objects

Rejects things, like food, by pushing away or scrunching
up face

Shows he doesn't feel well by exhibiting lethargy

Vocalizes to attract your attention

Relaxes when you sing to him

Tries to imitate speech sounds she hears

Grasps and looks closely at toys

Looks at pictures in books

Moves to quick music, is quieter with soft and slower music

Mouths many objects, so keep baby safe from hazards
(mouthing, sucking and chewing work the articulation
muscles)

Imitates simple hand movements

STAGES OF LANGUAGE DEVELOPMENT

3 to 6 months (continued):
Makes funny sounds with mouth and laughs at them
Understands a firm "No!"

By 6 months –
Responds to own name
Waves "bye-bye"
Listens when she hears her own name
Grasps toys
Prefers some colors, usually red and blue

6 months to 1 year:

Looks to where you point
Points to objects and holds them up to show people
Turns when you call her name
Attends to short stories
Helps you turn pages of cardboard books
Points to pictures in a book
Imitates many speech sounds and syllables
Turns, points, or otherwise responds to names of
    familiar objects and people: cup, bottle, juice, car,
    daddy, ball, Auntie
Responds to simple phrases: "Come on," "Want
    some juice?"
Likes baby games like patty-cake and peek-a-boo
Shakes head "no"
Uses body language to communicate
Attempts to find things hidden under a cloth or blanket
Hands a toy to someone to ask them to play with him
Responds to "Look at that" and "Look at the ____"
Makes "raspberry" sound with lips
Opens and closes her mouth when watching you eat

STAGES OF LANGUAGE DEVELOPMENT

6 months to 1 year (continued):
Likes to look at self in the mirror
Answers simple questions with sounds or body language
Shows frustration or anger if someone takes his toy
Moves with the rhythm of music
Stares at things and keenly observes
Stares at other children but does not interact
Becomes anxious with unfamiliar people
Points to objects named in picture book
Recognizes the names of family members
Claps hands
Can learn "baby signs"
Can learn turn taking (e.g. in a simple game like rolling a ball)
Looks for hidden objects

10 months –
Uses jargon (babbling with sentence prosody – intonation,
    stresses, pauses – so it almost sounds like sentences)
Joins in conversations with babbling or jargon
Understands about 40 words
Follows simple instructions like "Give me the cup"

11 months –
Points to object he wants as he vocalizes
Reacts differently to sounds in her native language vs.
    sounds in other languages

By 12 months –
Combines different syllables into one utterance
Uses objects meaningfully (e.g., stirring food with a spoon)
    while listening to caregiver's narration of the action
Says, "Mama," "Dada," "uh-oh!" and another few words,
    like "doggy" and "up"

STAGES OF LANGUAGE DEVELOPMENT

1 year to 18 months:

Understands (receptive vocabulary) about 100 words

Begins supporting words with gestures

Names pictures in books and points when you name them

Attends to longer stories

Turns pages of book

Turns book right side up

Brings book to adult to read it

May look very serious as you read to her

Makes animal noises

Uses 2-word utterances consistently like "more juice," "daddy come," "no bed"

Follows 1-step directions like "Pet the kitty" or "Get your cup"

Asks some questions, like "what that?"

Points to some body parts you name

Responds to simple questions like "Where's mommy?" and "Do you want more?"

Laughs at words she makes up herself

Expresses emotions broadly (loud laughter, tantrums, jumping up and down)

Sometimes consciously ignores requests of adults

May pass toys to another child, but still does not play with others

Listens to other children talk to each other

Tries to sing along with you

Uses some imagination in play

Listens to caregiver talking about baby's actions

Has an expressive vocabulary of 10 to 20 words by 16 months

STAGES OF LANGUAGE DEVELOPMENT

18 months to 2 years:

Expresses 50 words or more (expressive vocabulary) at 18 months, but may understand 300

Likes to join in singing songs

Joins in on predictable phrases in story books

Names many familiar objects in story books

Imitates adult hand movement (pointing to words and pictures) with story books

Fills in the next predictable word in story when adult pauses

"Reads" books to dolls or stuffed animals

Protests and/or corrects when adult skips words or mis-reads a book

Relates objects in books to real life (bear, truck, etc.)

Chooses book based on interest (doctor's office, taking a nap, etc.)

Mimics actions mentioned in books

Points to pictures to ask for the word (e.g., "Dat?")

Begins to use conversational conventions like asking and listening to answers

Uses many 2-word utterances (Daddy car, more juice, big ball, want milk) and some 3- and 4-word utterances

Uses words to ask for what she wants

Focuses on play for longer periods of time

Becomes frustrated when you don't understand him

Begins to play and share with other children

Often sticks her tongue out while concentrating on something

Uses most consonants and vowels in speech, but might mispronounce some

Copies many things you do

"Dances" to familiar music

Talks about some past events

STAGES OF LANGUAGE DEVELOPMENT

18 months to 2 years (continued):

Recognizes photos of herself

Listens to conversations and sometimes repeats words
heard (be careful of what you say)

By 2 years –

Has a receptive vocabulary of about 500 words

Has an expressive vocabulary about 200 words

Learns about 9 words per day (63 per week!)

Asks lots of questions

Uses imaginative play

2 to 3 years:

Speaks more clearly so he is understandable, especially to
people familiar with him (50 – 75% intelligible)

Uses quickly developing vocabulary for people, places,
things and actions

Understands 2-step directions like "Get your book, then sit
on the couch."

Talks about things not immediately present

Frequently asks, "What's that?" (Maybe "Whassat?" or
"Whaddat?") to learn new words

Listens to stories enthusiastically

Enjoys hearing the same stories over and over again

Asks questions about a story being read

Shows two books that have similar topics

Reenacts scenes from stories when playing

Starts using the suffix *-ing* ("Doggie runn*ing*")

Repeats many more words and sounds

Makes noises during pretend play, like imitating sounds of
trucks, babies or animals

Uses some prepositions like *in, on* and *under*, then *beside*
and *between*

STAGES OF LANGUAGE DEVELOPMENT

2 to 3 years (continued):

Asks "Why?" and even "Who," "What," and "Where," then listens attentively to answers

Overgeneralizes grammatical structures like the past tense morpheme *-ed* (drink*ded*, com*ed*, do*ed*)

Uses comfort objects (a favorite blanket, thumb sucking)

Enjoys simple conversations with adults and other children

Uses pronouns *I, you,* and *he*

Uses more language in imaginary play

Verbalizes toilet needs

Tells some personal information, like his name and age

Matches colors

Knows the difference between today and tomorrow

Asks the meaning of unfamiliar words

Recites some nursery rhymes

Recognizes details in picture books

Plays meaningfully with toys like dolls and trucks

Imitates vocal quality of different people in pretend play (you will recognize yourself in this)

Often speaks with loud voice

Sometimes omits final consonants in words

Appreciates being able to make choices

Turns pages of a book at the right point

Sorts objects by shape

By 3 years –

Has a receptive vocabulary of over 1000 words

Has an expressive vocabulary of about 250 words

Uses much more prosody (stresses, pauses, intonation) in speech

Speaks in phrases and sentences of 3 to 4 words

Switches from one topic to another in conversation

Makes up simple stories from imagination

STAGES OF LANGUAGE DEVELOPMENT

3 to 4 years:

Speaks with 80% intelligibility
Answers simple "Who," "What" and "Where" questions
Talks about events (current, past and future)
Understands and uses some color and shape words
Uses pronouns, but may be inconsistent: *I* vs. *me, her* vs. *she*
Uses some 6-word sentences
Uses contractions (*can't, don't, isn't,* etc.)
Plays with rhyming words: "kitty-bitty," "shoe-boo"
Uses some plural words: *toys, kitties, tables*
Asks "How" and "When" questions
Uses more past tense, but still with errors: "Mommy goed
   to the store"
Retells parts of a story
Understands object functions
Follows 2 – 3 step commands
Uses language to express emotion: "I'm mad!"
Tells 2 events in chronological order
Copies a circle
Copies and draws some easy alphabet letters (like O, C and V)
Attempts to write her own name
Writes "mock words," strings of letters that aren't real
   words
Tells about a picture she has drawn – does not just label it

By 4 years –
Has a receptive vocabulary of about 5,000 words
Has an expressive vocabulary of about 2,000 words
Uses *he* and *she* correctly

STAGES OF LANGUAGE DEVELOPMENT

4 to 5 years:

Understands "yesterday," "today" and "tomorrow"

Understands some order words like "first" and "last"

Follows 3-step directions: "Put your book away, get your water and sit with Grandma."

Understands most of what others say

Speaks very clearly (but might have some common articulation errors)

Uses future tense: "Jason will be here Sunday"

Has conversations that make sense, with turn-taking

Says the alphabet, recognizes and names most letters

Recites numbers 1 – 10, recognizes and names most when pointed to

Counts objects to 5

Uses longer, more complex sentences with more than one subject and verb, but still makes some grammatical errors

Calms friends who are upset

Copies a triangle, circle and cross

Enjoys jokes by 4 years

By 5 years –

Tells name, address and phone number

Is appropriate in conversations

Draws pictures with several items and a background

Plays both alone and with others

Points to Remember About Stages of Language Development:

➢ Your child's language development depends on you.

➢ Children learn language by being in a language-rich environment.

➢ Language is comprised of five major characteristics:

- ◆ **Phonemes** – the sounds of any language
- ◆ **Morphemes** – meaningful parts of words
- ◆ **Syntax** – sentence formulation and word order
- ◆ **Semantics** – vocabulary, ideas and meaning
- ◆ **Pragmatics** – the social use, purpose or intent of language

➢ As your child develops he becomes more aware (met-alinguistic awareness) of these aspects of language so he can use language for reading and writing, and for speaking well.

➢ Many parts of the brain are associated with speech and language, and you can stimulate these areas by providing the right kinds of activities for your child.

➢ You can keep track of your child's speech and language development by being aware of developmental milestones and by observing your child's attempts at communication every day.

➢ Your child doesn't need fancy toys, games or programs. Your child needs you as a model of speech and language and as an expert at encouraging communication and learning.

➢ Helping your child to develop language will be an absolute JOY for your child – and for YOU.

Great toys for babies and toddlers:

Soft storybooks

Rattles

Mobiles

Plastic building blocks

Plastic stacking rings

Shape puzzles with handles

Soft play mat

Unbreakable, easy grip mirror

Wooden animal puzzles

Wooden shape puzzles

Wooden or plastic cubes

Plastic nesting cups

Large plastic rings

Stuffed animals and snuggle toys

Wind-up music toys

Small plastic toy animals

Baby dolls

Dolls with easily removable clothes

Dollhouse

Pull toys with wheels

Plastic alphabet play mat or puzzle with bright colors

Plastic or wooden train with lots of train cars

Jack-in-the-box

Recordings of animal noises

Recordings of children's songs

Crayons and paper

Sand and water tray

Play-Doh of different colors

Peg board with wooden hammer

Toy telephone

Bath toys

Plastic cups, saucers and spoons

Toy musical instruments

Shape sorters

Category sorters

Toy cars and trucks

Various containers with lids

Plastic people toys showing various jobs

Toy tools

Arts and crafts materials: crayons, white and colored paper, child scissors, glue, cardboard

Child's table and chairs

Sit-on pedal toy

Plastic bat and ball

Soft rubber and inflatable balls

SHARING THE JOY

Here are some easy, but very important, ways to start your baby on a course of developing amazing language skills. Some of them will be repeated in later chapters with explanations of how they will enhance each aspect of language. For now, though, just enjoy your baby and watch him or her grow.

- ♥ Talk to your baby.

- ♥ Use various tones of voice.

- ♥ Use good eye contact and put your face very close to his.

- ♥ Use vivid facial expressions.

- ♥ Sing songs to your baby, especially songs with repetition, like "Old MacDonald Had a Farm."

- ♥ Respond to her sounds.

- ♥ Soothe your baby and take crying seriously.

- ♥ Try to figure out what her different sounds mean.

- ♥ React to her body language.

- ♥ Reflect his feelings with facial expressions and intoned phrases.

- ♥ Tickle your baby playfully.

- ♥ Sing action songs like "This Little Piggy" while playing with her.

- ♥ Provide rattles and toys that make sound.

- ♥ Let him play toy musical instruments, including using everyday objects to make music and rhythm.

- ♥ Recite rhymes and sing rhyming songs.

- ♥ Encourage listening by saying, "Listen – I wonder what that is," and then going to find the source of the sound.

- ♥ Attach mobiles and brightly colored toys to his crib.

- ♥ Give him toys of different textures.

- ♥ Show pleasure and enthusiasm when your baby is cooing and looking at you.

- ♥ Pause long enough for your baby to babble a response to you – as if you are having a conversation with her.

- ♥ Ask questions of your baby, even if she can't respond.

- ♥ Teach attention skills by ringing a little bell in different parts of the room to have your baby turn toward the sound.

- ♥ Read stories to your baby from early infancy and watch her attend to your face while on your lap and to the pictures you point to in the book.

- ♥ Play Peek-a-Boo games, hiding your face behind your hands and then reappearing.

- ♥ Help him search for things under clothing, blankets or pillows, asking, "Where do you think the _____ is?"

- ♥ Match your expression to hers to draw her interest to facial expressions and body language.

- ♥ Play different kinds of music to him, some soft and gentle, some more lively, and "dance" with him to the rhythm.

♥ Chat with your baby about people, objects and events in the home and during outings.

♥ Use facial expressions to make your baby laugh and tune in to your body language.

♥ Seat your baby so she can see your face when you talk to her and imitate her sounds.

And mostly – Be amazed by the ability of this little person to take all this in and to thrive on communication!

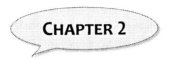

CHAPTER 2

Articulation and Phoneme Development: Making Sounds, Syllables and Words

Phonemes are the spoken sounds of any language. English is rather phoneme dense, containing about 40 phonemes, while other languages, like Spanish, have many fewer. Babies in all cultures produce and learn the phonemes they hear in their environment. Many languages also have a written version that is based on the sounds of the language, but not all languages do.

The act of speaking, for which your baby is preparing, is really quite remarkable. During speech, the brain signals the muscles of the lips, jaw, vocal cords and lungs to contract and relax at an extraordinarily quick pace, about eight phonemes per second. That's eight distinct sounds in one second! Think about that the next time you speak. In fact, say something out loud right now. Say your own name and be conscious of what your lips, tongue, teeth, jaw, vocal cords and lungs are doing. It's truly an incredible feat. Now think about what it takes to have a conversation!

How do babies develop the ability to make the sounds they need for speaking?

Preparation for speech actually begins months before birth. Babies are born with a good sense of hearing. Yes, babies do hear even before they're born, and they are born with a remarkable ability to discriminate sounds. In fact, fetuses can hear sounds around 18 weeks after conception. They hear their mother's voice, music, environmental sounds, etc. Mothers report that their fetus also responds to loud or high-pitched music and sounds, though not much to conversations, which are relatively quiet. Newborns, however, do respond to their mother's voice, so there is some recognition of it that begins before birth. Newborns can even hear the difference between phonemes, like the "p" sound and the "b" sound. Studies have shown that they will pause in sucking when the phoneme changes.

Infants can also discriminate sounds in their own language from sounds in other languages. Then by about 12 months they are most interested in phonemes produced by their caregivers. And babies not only listen, but they watch us very closely – essentially reading our lips. In fact, research has shown that babies will usually turn away from videos in which a person's lips are not in sync with their words. They know what language sounds like – and even what it looks like!

Infants begin practicing speech and language at birth, so the first year is crucial in this development. Infants' sounds are produced by the parts of their mouths used for sucking, eating and fussing. Babies make all kinds of sounds, and sounds begin with breathing. So having good lung power is important. Sometimes people joke about a baby who cries loudly as having great lungs, but, in fact, crying is a very important part of speech development, and the way a baby cries or giggles is the beginning of her use of language for communication.

Babies are quite different from toddlers and young children in the way their mouths and throats function. Babies are able to continue to breathe while nursing because of the position of the larynx (part of the throat containing the vocal cords). Later, the larynx drops in position to leave more room in the mouth and throat for speech. You will be able to watch your baby change physically as he becomes ready for speech.

There are many physiological reasons, other than those noted above, for speech sounds to develop the way they do, in a certain order. For instance, because infants usually lie on their back with their tongue hanging back in their mouth, the first speech sounds are often /k/ and /g/, which are sounds produced at the soft palate, in the back of the mouth. This part of the mouth is also used for sucking, so babies practice with it a lot. When parents imitate these baby sounds, they encourage baby to continue to "talk." In fact, a whole "conversation" can, and should, be started around the baby's sounds.

Baby: bababababoobooboo

Mom: Bababababoobooboo! Oh, my goodness! What a lot to say about being changed! I have a nice, clean diaper for you.

Baby: eeeoooweeeah

Mom: I know! Eeeoooweeeah! I think you really like this. Now here comes the powder!

It will seem as if your baby is developing actual speech pretty quickly. By about 4 months, after getting quite a bit of experience with crying, cooing and babbling, infants are better at manipulating their oral muscles and vocal cords, even being able to both shout and whisper. After about six months, your baby will have fun practicing strings of sounds he hears in the language of his family, usually in the form of syllables. You might hear "pipipipipi" or "ababababab," and, of course, the extra special "mamamama" and "dadada." Then you and Dad will get so excited ("She called me mama!") that you will call every family member with the news. Although this first "word" was just coincidence as she was practicing making sounds (sorry, Mom), when Mom begins referring to herself as "mama" and gets excited whenever baby repeats it, baby will learn it and use it spontaneously to actually mean "mama." At this point it has become a real word, even though it started as random phoneme syllables.

By about 10 months of age infants even babble with the prosodic features (stresses, pauses and intonation patterns) of phrases and sentences. Your baby will begin saying strings of various syllables with the prosody of statements, questions and commands, like "Abawamina?" and "Babagooooda!" He will have so much control over his vocal mechanisms that it will sound like real talking! So during the first year of life your baby is working very hard to become capable of pronouncing all the words he will need to communicate with you and with others.

How are all those sounds actually produced?

Sounds are produced by a combination of *place, manner* and *voicing*.

Place is the place in the mouth where the sound is produced. Our articulators are our tongue, teeth, lips and jaw. When we vary the positions of each, we can produce different sounds (phonemes). When speech-language pathologists and linguists note the sounds a child is making, they use slashes // to show that these are phonemes, not letters.

The following information is not absolutely necessary for you to know, but you might find it interesting. The letters within slashes // are sounds (phonemes). Most phonemes are written as letters of the alphabet, so you will know what they sound like. But some are not. Brackets [ ] are used here to indicate the way the phonemes would sound if you were to read them in English.

Try this: Produce each of these sounds as you read the descriptions to really understand how they are produced. Think about your articulators (lips, tongue, teeth, jaw) as you make the sounds.

- **Labio-dental (lip-teeth):** Sounds produced with the bottom lip and top teeth (/f/, /v/)

- **Inter-dental (between teeth):** Sounds produced with the tongue between the teeth (/θ/ and /ð/) ["soft" and "hard" "th"]

- **Alveolar (near the alveolar ridge):** Sounds produced with the tongue behind or touching the top front teeth, near the bumpy alveolar ridge (/s/, /z/, /ʃ/ [sh], /ʒ/ [zh as in "pleasure"], /n/, /t/, /d/, /l/, /dʒ/ [j], /tʃ/ [ch])

- **Palatal (near the hard palate):** Sounds produced with the tongue humped up near the hard palate, the roof of the mouth (/r/, /j/ [y])

- **Velar (at the velum):** Sounds produced with the tongue touching the soft palate (velum), behind the hard palate, in front of where the uvula hangs down (/k/, /g/, /ŋ/ [ng])

- **Glottal (in the glottis):** produced only from the opening between the vocal cords, the glottis (/h/)

The **manner** in which a phoneme is produced describes how the breath flows through the mouth and what **kind** of sound it makes. (popping, friction, nasal, etc.)

- **Stops or Plosives:** The air is stopped by the tongue or lips and then exploded (/p/, /b, /t/, /d/ and others)
- **Fricatives** and **Sibilants:** The air is restricted, thus causing friction (/f/, /s/, /v/ and others)
- **Nasals:** The air is expelled only through the nose (/m/, /n/ and /ŋ/ [ng])
- **Vowels:** The air is not stopped or constricted, but is produced only by placement of the tongue. The tongue is either high, low, back, front or in the middle of the mouth (/i/ [ee], /a/ [ah], /u/ [oo] and others)
- **Glides, Liquids** or **Semivowels** because they are more like vowels, not restricting the air (/l/, /r/, /j/ [y] and /w/)

The third aspect of phoneme production is called **voicing**. Sounds are either voiced or voiceless (unvoiced). During production of **voiced** phonemes the vocal cords vibrate and make sound (/b/, /d/, /l/, /z/ and many others), whereas **voiceless/unvoiced** phonemes are produced only with air flow (/p/, /k/, /s/, /f/ and many others). If you put your hand on your throat while producing different speech sounds, you will be able to feel the vibration with **voiced** sounds, but not with **voiceless** sounds.

Why does my child have difficulty pronouncing some sounds? Will she grow out of this?

A common reason why a child might substitute one sound for another, like saying "thun" instead of "sun," is that the inter-dental "th" sound is easier to pronounce than the alveolar

/s/. The brain knows, however, that both are fricative sounds, so acoustically they are very similar. In fact, the substitution doesn't make any difference in meaning. The remarkable human brain just knows that some phonemes sound pretty much alike, so the easier ones to pronounce can be substituted for the more difficult ones. Usually sound substitution is not a problem, as long as the child's speech is understandable, and he will soon learn and use the correct pronunciation of the phoneme.

Your child is good at choosing which sounds to substitute because his brain is very good at classifying speech sounds. It is probably more accurate than yours or his teacher's. Once we know how to spell, our perception of sounds in words changes. For example, we hear the /l/ phoneme at the end of the word "hall," but in fact it is quite different from the phoneme at the beginning of the word "like." A final /l/ is an **allophone** of /l/, which means that it is classified as /l/, but it is produced in a different place in the mouth and sounds somewhat different. Many adults don't hear the difference because we know that it is spelled with a double "l." Children's brains often hear the actual sounds, not the sounds we think we hear.

More About Speech Sound Production

Spelling changes the way we hear sounds. Say the word "top" and then the word "kitten." Did you notice that the "t" sound in each word is different? Now say "pot" and notice that the "t" is hardly pronounced at all. Try "stop" and notice that the "t" sounds more like a "d." Now say "stop" and "sdop." Do you hear any difference? We think we

---

59

hear certain sounds, but often those are not the sounds we are actually producing.

Speech sound production is actually a very complex process, so sequencing phonemes is no easy task for your child. Experiment with a few words as you read this section in order to understand the complexity of the speech sound system. You might wonder how complex pronouncing one phoneme, like /b/, can be. Well, all of the following actions occur within a split second: a person exhales, activates his vocal cords, puts his lips together, stops the air flow, and then pushes it out. Now say a word that begins with /b/, like "bicycle," and think about the process of articulation for each phoneme in the word. Your tongue is moving to many different areas of your mouth and your vocal cords are vibrating, and then not vibrating, then vibrating with each voiced sound, at incredible speed.

If your child has multiple articulation errors by age 3, so that her speech is difficult to understand, it is wise to take her to a speech-language pathologist for an evaluation. You can also do an informal assessment yourself. Do an audio recording of your child saying at least 100 words. Then have an unfamiliar listener write down all the words that can be understood. Have them put a line on the paper for each word that cannot be understood. Divide the number of words understood by the total number of words spoken. This will give you a percentage of intelligibility. Here are the general guidelines:

- 2-year-old should be 50% intelligible
- 3-year-old should be 75% intelligible
- 4-year-old should be 100% intelligible

That means that a 4-year-old whose words can only be understood 50% of the time has an articulation delay of about two years. "Intelligible" does not mean that every sound is produced perfectly; it means that every word can be understood.

Of course, many of these articulation difficulties are normal during a child's language development. A two-year-old commonly leaves off some final consonants ("ki" for "kiss") or internal syllables ("e-phant" for "elephant") and omits one consonant in a blend ("top" for "stop," "bu" for "blue," "kool" for "school"), but it gets better and better as the child approaches school age. By the time a child enters kindergarten his speech should be easy to understand, although he may still have a few common sound substitutions. Of course, there are specific words that are more difficult to pronounce, even for adults, but that is different from always substituting a "th" for an "s" or a "w" for an "r." Most five-year-olds, however, exhibit no continual speech sound errors at all.

When should my child be able to pronounce all speech sounds?

The chart on the next page shows the ages of acquisition of phonemes for boys and girls. These are the ages at which approximately 90% of children correctly produce the sound. The sounds in parentheses are the way we would usually spell them in English if different from the phonetic alphabet. A dash before a sound (–l) means the sound is at the end of the word or syllable. A dash after a sound (l–) means the sound is at the beginning of a word or syllable.

Age of Acquisition		Phonemes Written Sound ( )	Example Words
Girls	Boys		
3-0	3-0	m, h, w, p, b	mop, house, wet, pot, bat
3-6	3-0	n	not
3-0	3-6	d	dog
3-6	3-6	k, f-	key, cat, fun
4-0	3-6	t	top
3-6	4-0	g	go
4-0	5-0	j (y-)	yes
4-0	5-6	tw, kw (qu)	twin, queen
4-6	7-0	ð (th)	these
5-6	5-6	-f, v	off, laugh, very
5-0	6-0	l-	love
5-6	6-0	pl, bl, kl (cl), gl, fl	play, blue, clean, glass, floor
6-0	8-0	θ (th)	think
6-0	7-0	ʃ (sh), tʃ (ch), dʒ (j), -l	ship, chin, jump, hall
7-0	7-0	ŋ (ng), s, z, sp, st, sk, sm, sn, sw, sl, skw (squ), spl	sing, see, zebra, spin, stop, skin, small, snail, sweet, sleep, square, splash
8-0	8-0	-ɚ (er, or, ur), r-, pr, br, tr, dr, kr (cr), gr, fr	father, work, hurt, red, prize, brown, tree, drink, cream, green, from
9-0	9-0	θr (thr), spr, str, skr (scr)	three, sprain, string, scream

Figure 3: Chart adapted from Smit, A.B, Hand, L., Freilinger, J.J., Bernthal, J.E. & Bird, A. (1990). *Journal of Speech and Hearing Disorders*, 55, 779 – 798.

What kinds of articulation errors might my child make?

Here are the types of articulation difficulties children may exhibit:

Sound Substitutions – Usually sounds produced in the same manner and with the same voicing, but produced in a different place (like th/s [thun/sun]; th/z [cra<u>th</u>y/crazy]; w/r [wabbit/rabbit]; w/l [wike/like]; y/l [yunch/lunch]; t/k [tat/cat]; d/g [dood/good])

Phonemic Distortions – Not an English sound, but a distortion of the sound (like a lateral lisp: the air escapes over the sides of the tongue rather than through the front, like Daffy Duck in cartoons)

Allophones – Classified as the same phoneme, though pronounced slightly differently (like a /l/ at the beginning of a word that is pronounced as it would be at the end of a word); you recognize the sound, but it is pronounced just a little differently

Coarticulation Differences – Pronouncing phonemes in a sequence that, because of difficulty of pronunciation, often changes or omits some phonemes (like pronouncing "February" as "Febuary" or "animal" as "aminal")

Oral Motor Planning Difficulty – Difficulty with control of articulators; can be observed by having the child imitate sounds and oral movements (see more about this in Appendix A: Childhood Apraxia of Speech)

We usually take for granted our ability to produce words and sentences automatically, but it is, as was just explained, an incredibly complex sequence of movements. The more practice a baby gets at imitating sounds and words, the easier it will be for him to speak and to be aware of differences in words. It is well worth the effort to help your baby practice, practice, practice. Have fun encouraging your baby to play with sounds, and to imitate speech sounds, silly sounds, and funny tongue/lip/face movements. This is all very important preparation for speech.

SHARING THE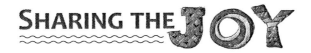

- ♥ Stick out your tongue a number of times to see if your baby will imitate your movements.

- ♥ Respond to your baby's sounds by imitating them while making happy facial expressions.

- ♥ Let her blow saliva bubbles to strengthen her lip muscles.

- ♥ When your baby is babbling, hold her up near your face, but don't look at her – then look into her eyes and hear how she "talks" even more to you.

- ♥ Practice all kinds of oral movements (protruding and retracting lips, waggling your tongue back and forth, tracing your lips with your tongue, sipping through a straw to make noise, etc.) as a game with your child – this will also demonstrate to you his oral motor ability.

- ♥ Speak clearly, sometimes emphasizing some sounds in words, to get your toddler used to listening for speech sounds.

- ♥ When you tell your toddler the names of objects and people, have him watch your mouth as you pronounce the words so he can imitate your movements.

- ♥ Teach tongue twisters to your 3 year old (and older), but be patient and start slowly, so he will see it as an enjoyable challenge.

- ♥ Read books with rhymes or funny words (Dr. Seuss, Shel Silverstein, etc.) and have fun focusing on the sounds of language as you read them to your child.

♥ If your 4-year-old consistently substitutes one sound for another in words (like "lellow" rather than "yellow"), try to figure out what your articulators (lips and tongue) are doing when you pronounce the sound, and once a day show your child how to do it, sometimes using a mirror for reinforcement.

♥ Here is something challenging, but fun to try. Go through the English consonants (starting at the beginning of the alphabet) and figure out which consonants are produced in these places in the mouth. Don't forget about the phonemes that are spelled with more than one letter, digraphs like sh, ch and th. Write them on the lines. Do it with your 4- or 5-year-old as an excellent metalinguistic activity! The number of consonants for each place of articulation is in parentheses. The answers are on page 86.

Bilabial (4)_____

Labio-dental (2)_____

Lingua-dental (Interdental) (2)_____

Alveolar (10) _____

Palatal (2) _____ **Velar** (3)_____ **Glottal** (1)____

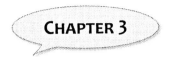

CHAPTER 3

Learning New Words (Vocabulary) and Meanings: Semantic Development

Semantics is the study of meaning; *vocabulary* is a way to understand and express meaning. You may have heard someone say, "It's a matter of semantics." This generally means that two or more people use a different word for a concept, or express an idea somewhat differently. The semantics of oral, written, or signed language, as it is used in this guide, is what the speaker, writer or signer really means.

In the Form – Content – Use diagram in Chapter 1: The Basics, it is labeled "Content" because it is the content of what we are communicating. It is what we are talking about or writing about. But, as the diagram illustrates, it converges and overlaps with Form (phonology/morphology/syntax) and Use (pragmatics).

Think for a moment about a situation in which you were misunderstood. You may have wondered how on earth the person completely misinterpreted what you were saying. Misunderstanding occurs frequently when one doesn't tune in to *how* something is said (vocal intonation, facial expression and body language) and to the intention of the speaker (pragmatics), in addition to understanding the meanings of the words.

Experiences in infancy set the foundation for vocabulary and semantic development. Babies and toddlers notice, think, categorize, wonder, and seek out new experiences. This is a crucial stage of brain development. Exploration plus interactions with the language of parents and caregivers are laying the foundation for the learning of concepts and the words to express them. Your baby will begin to develop a vocabulary during the second year of life, and this development will continue throughout his entire lifetime.

It has been well documented that most children who have a good vocabulary at age three have the vocabulary skills at ages nine and ten that lead to academic success. Children entering school with well-developed vocabularies are at a significant advantage for learning, especially when reading. When a child has an extensive vocabulary, it generally means that caregivers have taught him the names of things in his environment and have made language interesting, sparking the child's curiosity for words.

A child's vocabulary will grow by thousands of words through elementary and middle school, then through high school and for the rest of her life. If a child begins school with a fairly extensive vocabulary and is accustomed to focusing on new words every day (you will play a crucial role in this), by high school graduation this child will understand about 80,000 words!

How does vocabulary develop?

Just think of all the language a baby is hearing each day. It is certainly not unusual for mother and father to be talking to each other while sister is trying to get their attention and brother is talking on the phone while the TV is on in the background. Babies hear people talking all the time. Can you imagine what this sounds like to a baby? How does a baby pick out individual words from all this commotion going on?

Luckily, babies are born biologically ready to learn language by seeking regularities in the patterns of the language they hear around them. They are born wanting to hear language and wanting to learn how to use it themselves, so they tune in to conversations around them. They quickly discover what language sounds like, and they listen to it very carefully. They turn their heads toward voices. In fact (this is pretty remarkable), studies have shown that they even know when people are using the correct prosody (stresses and intonation) of their language. Your baby doesn't understand what the sentences *mean*, of course, but he knows how language *sounds.*

Baby's attention to prosody, and imitation of prosody, precedes understanding by quite a few months. She will most likely attend to sentences with regular stresses and pauses and not to "irregular" sentences because she is tuning in to speech patterns that she will soon be using herself.

Babies first perceive sentences as strings of intoned sounds, not as individual words. A baby might hear, "Ohmygoodnessyoureallylikethosecarrotstoday!" not perceiving or understanding, "Oh, my goodness. You really like those carrots today!" However, after hearing "carrots" a number of times while he is being fed carrots, he will be able to separate that set of sounds from the rest of the sounds and add meaning to it. Research has even suggested that when caregivers touch a baby, even at four months, these tactile cues may facilitate the baby finding individual words in continual speech. So there is some indication that early vocabulary may also be linked to caregiver-infant physical interaction.

When do babies begin to understand words?

Shortly after birth infants change their sucking behavior (either pausing their sucking or becoming more intense), their eye movement, and their head turning when they hear speech sounds. They do not yet perceive individual words within running speech, but they do begin learning vocabulary as early as 6 month of age, when they begin to look at objects named by caregivers. And although they are beginning to understand words, they usually don't speak their first word until around their first birthday.

You will be able to tell when your baby is able to understand the meaning of a word, even when it is spoken as part of a phrase. You will see that spark of recognition. When learning language, or anything else, babies' brains are constantly categorizing things into important and unimportant: the names of things that are important (mommy, daddy, kitty, juice) and events that make a difference to the baby (eating, bath time, nap time, riding in the car). Babies are hard at work categorizing words to make meaning of the language they hear. When you emphasize important words to your baby, watch for a smile, a head turn, or other signs of recognition.

Will my baby's first word be "mama"?

Your baby's first word will definitely be one that holds a lot of meaning for him, but it might not be *mama* or *dada*. Don't be surprised if it is the name of a pet (*Kiki*), an object (*poon* [spoon]) or an action (*up*). *Mama* and *dada* will follow very soon after. Remember that babies are producing the /m/ and /d/ sounds along with vowels while babbling, so it is inevitable that a *mama* or *dada* will be produced. If Mama or Dada are there to hear it, and then get excited and repeat it to baby, it is likely to become a favorite word – and perhaps the first word. So it is very possible that *mama* will be baby's first word!

What other words will my baby say early?

First words will be words that have most meaning to your baby: specific nouns and verbs, and words needed to express himself like *no, more, again, up* and *bye-bye*. He will also use words that contain the sounds that he finds easiest to produce, and this varies from child to child. If he finds it more difficult to produce the /m/ sound than the /d/ consistently, he will probably say *"Dada"* many more times than he will exclaim *"Mama!"*

Babies first understand words that they hear often and that are important to them, like *cup, dog, car* or *hat*. They enjoy listening to stories that repeat familiar words over and over in slightly different contexts, and they begin to recognize them as old friends. Eventually they understand the meanings of these words, and then they begin to use them themselves. Babies at six or seven months seem to know their own name, but even with their own name it is unclear whether they just recognize this string of sounds as familiar or if they actually know that these sounds refer specifically to them. Many months of preparation (developing receptive vocabulary) are necessary for baby to utter her first words.

Each baby also has a preferred type of expression. Some babies are more expressive of their wants and needs, thus using words like *no* and *more* often. Others enjoy labeling people and objects such as *juice, Kiki* and *doggie*. You will get to know your child's style quickly by just observing. Then you can use these types of words with your child to increase her vocabulary repertoire more quickly. Of course, your child will also be learning words and word combinations of all types as soon as she needs them.

Toddlers also overgeneralize words they use. They might use the word *dog* to mean all animals or *ball* to mean everything that's round. Still too young to have much of a vocabulary, it makes sense to use a word that is at least close to what they want to say. This is another remarkable example of how baby's brain works and how she is learning. She is able to categorize objects and actions at a very early age, and is then able to search her memory for a word that belongs in that category. Of course, when baby calls a cow a dog, Mommy will probably say, very gently, "No, Sally, that's a cow." Eventually she will learn it's a cow – but for now she is showing you how smart she really is.

Will I understand my baby's first words?

Your child's "first word," and subsequent words, must have certain characteristics to be considered "real" words: they must be uttered with intention and purpose; they must mean the same thing each time they are used; they must be pronounced the same way each time; and they must be spoken to mean the same thing in different contexts. Sometimes it takes some doing and quite a bit of observation to figure out just what baby means by his first words. Does "pay" (play) mean playing outside, being lifted into the air, or being tickled? All three? Only in one context? Only when wanting to play with Daddy? Baby might even forget the word when she wants to express herself in an emotional context. Sometimes it just takes too much energy to be emotional and verbal at the same time.

Should I be using sign language with my baby?

The book *Baby Signs* by Drs. Linda Acredolo and Susan Goodwyn (there are also other good books on this subject) illustrates how babies have an irrepressible need to communicate. Their research of 140 families showed substantial advantages to teaching babies to sign. According to their research, these babies were less frustrated, were able to communicate their needs, developed more advanced oral language skills, and even did better on intelligence tests. Many parents have reported that their babies enjoyed signing and that the babies' language developed well.

Baby signs are much more illustrative of what they stand for than are the signs of American Sign Language (ASL), and they are easier for babies to sign. For example, the sign for "fish" in ASL is wiggling one or both hands across the front of the body to demonstrate the swimming motion of a fish. A baby sign for fish, however, could be opening and closing the mouth with a popping sound, like a child might see a fish doing in a tank. The ASL sign for "airplane" takes quite a bit of dexterity to make the "Y" sign with three fingers, but a baby friendly sign might be just to raise arms out to the side, like wings. Of course, you can make up your own signs with your baby, as long as you both know what they mean. The object is to give your baby a way to communicate with you – even before she can talk.

Many parents are afraid that if they allow their baby to sign, the baby will become dependent on signing and will have no need to speak. In fact, though, mothers who are in tune with their babies' communication through signing are able to expand upon the signs and put baby's intention into words. For example, if a baby made the sign for "juice," Mom could say, "Oh, you want some more apple juice. Okay, I'll get you some." Once baby is successful at getting his needs met with signs, he, like Mom or Dad, will also begin to use words. Many language development experts believe that signing leads to early talking, because parents and caregivers who gesture with babies are more responsive to their non-verbal cues. So yes, signing is a great way to communicate with your baby.

How many words should my toddler be using?

Your baby's first words will begin between 9 and 12 months of age, and before your baby is two years old she will have a vocabulary of about 50 words and will begin combining them into 2-word utterances. After she is using between 50 and 100 words, her vocabulary will develop in leaps and bounds, and at age 4 she should have a vocabulary of about 5,000 words!

Of course, some children acquire vocabulary at a much faster rate than other children, and this is usually a result of hearing a variety of words at home or in child care, and having the opportunity for plenty of practice. It has also been shown that children who use their hands to gesture at an early age also develop vocabulary early, possibly because they are trying to communicate even before they have the words to use (also see the section on baby sign language above). So increasing the diversity of words used with your child, and also the gestures that are used with new words, are both important components of vocabulary development.

What are some typical milestones for vocabulary development?

You can determine whether your baby is developing the skills for learning vocabulary long before he utters his first word. For example, studies suggest that 7½-month-old babies who are able to pick out (with a head turn) individual words within a context have a greater expressive vocabulary at 24 months. So begin testing your baby's attention to sounds and words within the first few months. Babies who attend to words and imitate sounds early begin to use words earlier.

At eight or nine months we can see that not only do babies attend to words, but they actually intend to communicate. They begin to understand that their actions (the cause), is followed by being given what they want (the effect). So your baby will look at you, touch you and vocalize while pointing to an object (like a cookie) or to signal to you to continue playing the game (like tickle or knee bounce). Interestingly, though, at this age the baby initiates the pointing. Babies at this age don't look at something that you are pointing at; they are more likely to look at your finger than at the object. They usually don't look at an object to which you are pointing until the end of the first year, just around the time of their first word.

Although your baby will not begin speaking until she is about one year old, she will by this time understand (receptive vocabulary) about 50 words, words that she hears very frequently: juice, milk, spoon, kitty, doggie, car, bath, diaper, Mommy, Daddy, Sally, no, don't, uh-oh, etc.

At about 12 to 18 months she will understand that all things have a name, and she will become curious about these names. She will want to label everything. Of course, we are often not sure just what she is naming. For example, when she says "tree" she might mean the entire tree or just the leaves.

At 18 months your baby should be interested in words, and should be trying many of them out. Being able to name objects and actions allows your baby to more easily get his needs met and to experience another way of bonding with people. In fact, there is evidence that a vocabulary delay at 18 months to 24 months can lead to behavioral/emotional problems, very likely because of the frustration experienced by children not being able to communicate their desires and feelings in a socially appropriate way – through oral language. So learning to use words that are important to him is crucial to his social/emotional development.

At 18 to 24 months, when your baby is developing so much vocabulary, you can notice how he tunes in to new words. If you put four familiar objects (like ball, teddy, bottle and spoon) on a table along with an unfamiliar object (like your driver's license), and ask baby, "Where's the license?" he will probably look at it or touch it. Even though he might not know the word "license," he knows it is not a ball, teddy, bottle or spoon. The novelty of new words gets baby's attention, and if they're used frequently and seem important to baby, he'll learn them.

Between 24 and 36 months you will notice quite a spurt in the way your child expresses herself. Three-year-olds can talk about past and future, and have respectable conversations using more than 1000 words, and understanding many more. They also use a variety of nouns and verbs, as well as descriptive words, which seem quite sophisticated for their age: nice, want, need, touch, taste, know, think, now, later, many, pretzel, elephant, reindeer. It has been shown repeatedly that the quantity of spoken language, richness of vocabulary and complexity of sentences of mothers' (so also fathers' and caregivers') speech affects the rate at which children acquired productive vocabularies and ease of finding the right word for the situation.

What can I do to make sure my child is developing a good vocabulary?

First, while your child is still a baby, you can use "infant-directed" speech, a type of speech that is very sing-songy and somewhat high pitched. It sounds like something babies would like to listen to. When caregivers use infant-directed speech, it lets babies know that this message is for them, that this is their special time to learn language and to have a close interaction and communication with a caring adult. For instance, if Aunt Martha and baby Kevin are looking through a picture book together, the conversation with an 18 – 24-month old might go something like this:

Aunt Martha: Oh, look at what the bunny is doing!

Kevin: Bunny.

Aunt Martha: Yes. The bunny is going to hop over the little fence to get to the carrots.

Kevin: Hop!

Aunt Martha: That's right! Hop! Look at him hop over the fence. He wants to eat the carrots.

Were you reading this with a lot of sing-songy expression? Good!

Another way that infants learn meaning and develop vocabulary is in giving "joint attention" to objects with an adult. When you both look at the same object and you comment on it, an important part of language learning is being developed – practice with shared experiences. This can also be done while playing together using just sounds. For example, if you or baby knocks over some blocks, you can exclaim, "Uh-oh!" Or if you put too much baby food on the spoon, you might remark (with a lot of intonation), "Oh! My goodness!" Joint attention actually involves a number of steps: following the child's focus, initiating episodes of joint attention, engaging in turn-taking, and switching between initiating and responding to the child.

For this example, Sue is playing with her doll:

Mommy: Oh, you're holding Kathy so nicely.

Sue: Hold Katty.

Mommy: Yes. Can you rock Kathy? (pretend to be rocking a baby)

Sue: Wok Katty.

Mommy: That's right. She loves you to rock her like that. Rocking her might even put her to sleep.

Sue: Seep?

Mommy: Yes, Sue. You're rocking Kathy to sleep.

It's so important for parents and caregivers to talk to the baby throughout the day and evening. While getting dinner ready, Mother might comment, "Mommy's got to peel the potatoes. Look at the potato, Rebecca. I wonder how many I should make. I wonder if Daddy is going to be really hungry tonight. I'd better make an extra one just in case. I can peel them all and then keep them in the pot of water till Daddy gets home. Then we'll be all set to cook everything!"

Besides commenting on things around you, it is very important to follow your baby's lead, commenting on what he is interested in and interacting with him as if in a conversation. When parents follow the baby's lead at nine months, their babies at thirteen months have greater receptive vocabularies. On the other hand, when parents do not attend to what interests baby, and who change the topic, baby's vocabulary at thirteen months is smaller. It is similar with adults; we don't learn much and become less attentive if we are speaking to someone who keeps changing the topic. Some people might call this being "dissed." We don't like it, and neither do babies. Of course, sometimes we need to change the topic or attend to something else, as long as we don't do it all the time.

How will you know what your baby is interested in? Watch her. She will actually have a style of interests that you should be aware of. There are two major styles of vocabulary learners. Children whose first words are mostly labels of things (nouns) like "juice" and "doggy" are considered "referential" children. If the children's first words are action words (verbs) like "bye-bye" and "up," they are "expressive" children. This difference might be personal preferences of the children, or they might be the kinds of words parents use with them, like parents who label things all the time for baby, or parents who frequently use words of social interaction. In either case, notice your child's first words and continue to add to her repertoire.

Whichever type of vocabulary learner your child is, also be observant about his interests. If he gravitates toward action and motion, play "This Little Piggy,' "Tickle-Tickle," "Whoop-sy-Daisy," "All gone," or "Peek-a-Boo." If he is more of a "noun lover," play "Where's your (body part)?" or "What's this?" Either is fine. You will figure it out by watching your baby and letting him express himself in his own style.

Always be aware of the progress your child is making with vocabulary. You can observe this when your child begins to express "shades" of meaning. For example, consider how we as adults think about opposites. When we express concepts like "hot" and "cold" we usually have a concept of these ideas along a continuum that at one end is "hot," and at the other end is "cold." When toddlers are learning descriptive words like *hot* and *cold, big* and *little* or *fat* and *skinny*, they don't learn them as opposite pairs. They are more likely to say *not hot* than *cold* or *warm* because it takes more advanced cognitive development to understand the continuum, or progression, of the concept. It is similar with learning the names of colors. *Blue* can mean a variety of shades of blue. Don't expect your toddler to know *aqua*, but note when all of a sudden your child uses more specific words to express ideas. That's when you can really see the relationship between language and cognition.

Does my child's aptitude with sounds and sentences affect her vocabulary development?

Actually, the ability to rhyme and the knowledge of which sounds are in a word do seem to be closely related to vocabulary development. A young child's ability not only to interpret spoken language, but also to recognize when she has heard a new word, is a good predictor of early language development. This seems to be connected to her skill in hearing phoneme differences so she knows when she hears a new word.

There is also the interest of words that sound alike but have different meanings, like *stair* and *stare* (homonyms). This is especially true of words that are articulated correctly by the adult and not by the child (adult: right – write; child: wight –

wite). This similarity in phonemes might make the child focus on the new word with interest because it has an unexpected meaning.

The sentences your child hears and uses also affect vocabulary development. As was illustrated in the Form-Content-Use diagram, semantics, (content/ideas) is also expressed through syntax (sentence structure). Many sentences may contain the same words, but the order of those words and the way they are spoken determine the real meaning of the sentence. Everything conveys meaning: thoughts, intention, sounds, words, sentences, prosody, body language and facial expressions. So children who always have something to say, and who use a variety of sentence types, also learn the words they need to get their ideas across to others.

What else can I do to develop good vocabulary in my preschooler?

Once your child is in preschool or goes on frequent outings with you, a good way to encourage her to remember vocabulary is to have her use the new words to retell her experiences: a trip to the grocery store, driving to Grandma's, watching a movie, walking the dog. And, of course, one of the best ways to teach a preschooler new words is through books. Retelling a story is, to a child, retelling an experience.

Of course, some parents cannot often take their children on trips, to museums, to farms, or on other exciting excursions to learn new vocabulary and concepts about the world. Although it is difficult to discuss a sporting event when children don't know the word "athlete," teachers and parents can teach new concepts and vocabulary by using books, as well as daily experiences, as a "Virtual Field Trip" or "Vocabulary Visit." Then retelling the story or experience makes it even that much more memorable. It has been shown that preschoolers who learned new vocabulary from science books retained the target words at a significantly higher rate after retelling the content of the books. Words that are unfamiliar to your child can even be listed on paper or sticky notes and organized into categories (body parts, weather, the jungle, etc.), and then other books about those subjects can review, reinforce and expand the vocabulary. Since so much of our vocabulary is acquired from reading, anyway, not just from life experiences, this is a perfect way to experience the world!

Research has found that young children also need to be actively engaged during the reading of the book if they are to remember new words and to understand the multiple meanings of words. So reading aloud to your child while having a dialogue with her about the story, as well as repeating key words and ideas, is a good way to keep your child engaged. You should also be questioning, providing definitions and synonyms, giving examples, clarifying or correcting her responses, labeling, and even bringing attention to morphemes, pointing out prefixes and suffixes and talking about what they mean. (This will be explained further in Chapter 4.)

When your child learns to read and write, he will also learn that word meaning affects spelling, and this will increase his vocabulary when he tries to figure out the meaning from the way the word is spelled. For example, you can "sell" things at your garage sale while you talk on your "cell" phone. Very often vocabulary and spelling go hand in hand. (Think about homonyms.) You can begin bringing attention to this with your preschooler so it will not be so confusing to him when he begins to write.

When your child is almost ready for kindergarten, you should also make her aware of ambiguous and figurative language. She might not really understand yet, but at least this awareness will prepare her to discover multiple meanings of words within a year or two. English contains so many ambiguous, multiple meaning words that we use every day, and we are usually not even aware that we are doing so. Dust the furniture could literally mean to put dust on the furniture, but it generally means to take dust off the furniture. If our alarm clock doesn't go off, we don't wake up on time. But literally it was off; it didn't go on. That's why we didn't wake up. Does "Turn right here?" mean we should turn here immediately, or that we should not turn left? Isn't English fun?

Of course, there are also personal differences among children which affect vocabulary development. For example, children who are shyer and not as eager to interact with others in social situations often lag in vocabulary acquisition. In this case, encouraging social skills might accelerate language development. Remember, however, that there is a range of normal development for all skills, so just continue to focus on new words and their meanings with your child so that he develops a love of language.

Will being in preschool affect my child's vocabulary development?

It depends upon the preschool and how attentive the teachers and staff are to the language needs of the youngsters. Studies have suggested that preschool children who are involved with more complex conversations with diverse vocabulary, even children who enter preschool with a lower vocabulary, will gain a greater expressive vocabulary by the time they are ready for school. But research has also indicated that the opportunity for meaningful conversations between children and adults are at a minimum in some preschool classrooms. You should be aware of how the staff at your child's preschool encourages language learning.

Some preschool classrooms have even set up "Conversation Stations" where children have an opportunity to talk, ask questions, get feedback on their oral language, and have close contact with adults who model appropriate language skills for them. In this way, language learning is systematically included in daily activities in addition to the language that is used throughout each day. Explicit instruction, repeated language experiences, and active engagement in these language experiences increases both vocabulary and understanding of narrative language regardless of the level of language proficiency a child brings to school. It is imperative that teachers of young children provide this instruction, for social language, reading comprehension, and a variety of types of academic language. So you need to choose a preschool that offers these rich language experiences to your child. There will be more information about choosing a preschool in Appendix B: Choosing a Preschool or Caregiver.

SHARING THE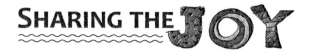

- ♥ Chat with your baby about people, objects and events in the home and during outside activities.

- ♥ Don't force her first words, but let them be the words she wants to say.

- ♥ Respond positively to each new word he adds to his vocabulary.

- ♥ Name everyday household objects.

- ♥ Name body parts and make a game of it.

- ♥ Give simple third party instructions like "Give the spoon to Teddy."

- ♥ Give instructions using prepositions: "Put the box under the table." "Put Teddy next to Aunt Jenny." "Which toy is between the truck and the boat?"

- ♥ Stress important words in your sentences, like prepositions. (I'm putting the dish <u>on</u> the table. Let's put the broom <u>in</u> the closet.)

- ♥ Give your toddler choices so he can practice naming what he wants.

- ♥ Discuss his art work with him, listening attentively to his descriptions.

- ♥ Encourage her to do things on her own, to be more independent when she wants to be – as long as she is safe (like putting on shoes, feeding herself, or completing an activity).

- ♥ Make up songs about daily tasks while doing them.

- ♥ Teach nursery rhymes, songs and poems a portion at a time.

- ♥ When looking at picture books, if the real object is in the room, point to it along with the picture of it.

- ♥ Modify part of a familiar story to encourage listening and memory.

- ♥ Have her use the new words to retell the situation where the words were initially experienced.

- ♥ Talk about stories you've read the day after you read them: "Remember when _(whatever happened)_ in the story about the fish?"

- ♥ Provide dress-up clothes to spark imagination and to practice being other people or grown-ups.

- ♥ Describe what is happening now, what he is doing, and what you are doing.

- ♥ Ask some clarification questions during his tales of events when he doesn't use enough detail. (What is his name? What was he having for a snack? Were you sitting together?)

- ♥ Expand your toddler's vocabulary by using synonyms (_huge_ instead of _big_, _delicious_ instead of _good_, _thrilled_ instead of _happy_).

- ♥ Point out differences in size, weight, color, etc. to build vocabulary, noticing small differences.

- ♥ Ask her to sort objects. ("Let's put the red ones here and the blue ones there. Can you put all the different birds in this box?")

♥ Give your child clues about objects new to her vocabulary: "It's the sweet liquid we pour over our pancakes."

♥ Explain the meaning of new words, like *frustrated* or *aqua.*

♥ Name items in a category and see if your child can name the category (animals, birds, food, furniture, weather, body parts, etc.).

♥ List words that are unfamiliar to your child on paper or sticky notes and organize them into categories.

Answers to phoneme placement exercise at end of Chapter 2: **bilabial** – p, b, m, w; **labio-dental** – f, v; **lingua-dental** – th, <u>th</u>; **alveolar** – s, z, l, n, t, d, sh, ch, zh, j; **palatal** – r, y; **velar** – k, g, ng; **glottal** – h

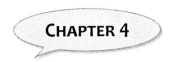

CHAPTER 4

Using Sentences:
Morphemes + Syntax = Grammar

Syntax is basically word order, but this definition greatly simplifies it. The formulation of sentences is actually an extraordinarily complex process. Those of us who do not have a problem representing our thoughts in sentences rarely think about it at all. It just happens automatically. When you have a thought that you would like to communicate to someone, you rarely have to decide upon how you are going to represent that thought linguistically. If you had to think about every sentence before it was spoken, you would hardly be able to speak at all. You might feel like a beginning French student who needs to take time to translate every sentence. That leads to very little language usage.

Morphemes are the smallest units of meaning in a language. Now what does that mean? It means that morphemes are root words, prefixes, suffixes, and the addition of tenses to words. You know that root words (like *stop* and *color*) have meaning. But we can also add something to *stop* to change its meaning. We can add *ed*, which means the action has already happened. (She *stopped* running) We can add a suffix to *beauty* (*ful*) so that it describes something that is full of beauty, or *beautiful*. So root words have meaning, and parts of words also have meaning.

Here are some examples of morphemes:

Root words – *stop, table, pretty, quick*

Prefixes – *un* (untie), *dis* (disappear), *auto* (automatic)

Suffixes – *ing* (walking), *ed* (played), *tion* (invitation), *s* (cats)

Present progressive tense – *ing* (painting)

Past tense – *ed* (climbed), *t* (slept)

Irregular verb tenses are also morphemes, but they change the word internally (come/came) rather than adding a suffix (stop/stopped).

Young children are just beginning to acquire morphemes that are attached to root words. They are learning the rules and using these morphemes to add meaning to sentences. Now, since language and thinking go hand in hand, you will know when your child is thinking about events that have already happened, or are going to happen, by the words he uses.

Later, when your child is in middle school and high school, teachers will be teaching him to recognize, understand and label morphemes. This plays an important role in learning to spell well and in being able to figure out word meanings. You can understand how knowing the meanings of prefixes and suffixes can help your child to increase his vocabulary – and metalinguistic awareness. So when your preschooler increases his use of morphemes, he's already on his way to academic success.

The use of syntax (sequencing words in order to convey specific ideas) and morphology (adding specific meaning to words) is what we call grammar. When we were young and our parents or teachers corrected our grammar, they were suggesting small changes, as many adults do. If we had not been speaking in sentences at all, however, they would have been much more concerned, and would have been happy for us just to make these small errors. So when we think about grammar, we usually think about a child not speaking "properly." Now you can think of grammar, though, as the usage of word order and word forms.

Is it difficult for children to learn to speak in sentences?

It is not difficult for most children because they are born with the capacity to acquire very complex language. Human beings' brains are "wired" for language. But when a brain is not wired properly for the acquisition of sentence structure, it causes multiple problems with oral and written language. Many children over four who don't speak very much might not just be "shy"; they might actually have difficulty formulating sentences. They might often use very short sentences and phrases because they are not able to express ideas in any other way. So learning to speak in sentences is not normally difficult, although the rules governing morphology and syntax are amazingly complex.

It is necessary for parents to understand that language cannot actually be taught to young children; it must be acquired. It can be corrected and fine-tuned, but not taught in its entirety. This is why it is imperative that parents and caregivers understand all aspects of language and create a language rich environment for children's brains to be exposed to and recognize patterns of words, phrases and sentences.

If a child has not developed the ability to formulate sentences in her early years, a parent, or even a speech-language pathologist, cannot effectively teach a child to use complex language. It is possible to train a child to use some simple sentences ("This is a cup." "This is a spoon.") with newly learned vocabulary, but children with no language cannot be taught to use the complex sentences that we use every day. That skill has to be acquired in the home and from caregivers. In fact, most children who are diagnosed with a language disability actually have a syntax disorder, which means they have difficulty understanding and/or expressing sentences.

To formulate sentences with good vocabulary, word choice and word order, and appropriate morphemes in a socially appropriate way, is an extremely complicated task. Do a little experiment here. Start thinking about a conversation you would like to have with someone. Now think of a possible sentence you might use in the conversation. (This is another use of language: rehearsing conversations and discussions or arguments.) For instance, you might say, "I don't care who asked you to stay late at work, you should have called to tell me what time you would be home." That's a 24-word sentence that most of us would have no trouble formulating. Can you imagine trying to teach a child how to do that? We think a thought, and we immediately and spontaneously translate that thought into oral utterances with the exact structure of a specific language. Amazing!

Many children with language problems utter very short phrases, one for each thought, as they try to narrate or explain something. These short utterances are spoken in the order of the child's individual thoughts. For instance, a language delayed child might say, "I have homework. Tonight. No TV. My mother say," instead of, "My mother told me I have to do my homework instead of watching TV tonight." Do you now see how terrifically complicated this is – the process of expressing thoughts all together in a grammatically appropriate, complex sentence?

How do sentences begin?

Let's start your child's first words. Words are either *content* words or *function* words. The content words are those that carry the content, or meaning, in a sentence. The function words are those that function as part of our grammar, but carry little meaning. Which type do you think your child will learn first?

Of course he will learn those words that carry the most meaning, the content words.

Content words are nouns, verbs, adjectives, adverbs and question words (who, what, when, where, why). They are the words spoken by young children who are just acquiring language: *mama, dada, juice, milk, cookie, up.* They are the words that carry the content, or the message, of the utterance. Language with only content words is called "telegraphic" speech because when we used to send telegrams, we would pay by the word. So only the content, or important, words would be used.

Function words are words such as articles, conjunctions, auxiliary verbs and prepositions. Their function is to add grammar to sentences. For example, the preposition *of* has 21 definitions in the *Merriam-Webster Dictionary* (online), and none has much real content; but we need "of" to make our sentences grammatical. Articles (the, a, an) also have no content; they let us know that a noun or noun phrase is next. Would a child's first word ever be *the*? Of course not. It has no meaning, and it really isn't needed for meaning.

How do babies figure out which sounds are "words"?

Can you imagine how difficult it must be for a baby to figure out where one word ends and another begins when she hears "Doyouthinkwecanstopatmymothersonthewayhome?" When we hear sentences, we don't have any difficulty understanding the *segmentation* of the sentence: individual words in the sequence. How do babies know where one word ends and another begins? Well, since your baby's brain is a very sophisticated pattern detecting device, it picks up on patterns of frequently heard strings of sounds that are often spoken a little louder than other sounds (content words vs. function words) within a context. Mommy says, "Doyouwantsome*juice*?" while holding up the bottle of apple juice time and time again. "Juice!"

How do babies begin to combine words?

When baby is learning his first words, he is actually able to communicate with those words pretty well. Since he can only utter one word at a time, he has to express a whole thought with that one word. These utterances are called "holophrases" (whole phrases in one word) and are used to comment or to make a request. This is the precursor to sentence formulation. Your child might yell, "Ball!" when his ball rolls under the chair. Because of his prosody (volume and stress), you know he's anxiously commanding you to do something – to get his ball out from under the chair – and that something has happened that is upsetting. Since prosody develops in the babbling stage, it makes sense that it now is used with words to make meaning and intent pretty clear. Now he's really talking, and almost ready to begin speaking in sentences.

Then, after baby has a vocabulary of about 50 words, she begins to combine words into simple, 2-word utterances. Your child will have words that are important to her – nouns, verbs, and some others. For example, the word *more* is usually important to little ones because they often ask for *more*. This might become a word for other words to be attached to in 2-word utterances: *more* milk, *more* juice, *more* hug, *more* up. The words that are used with them are the new vocabulary words she is learning every day. Another favorite word might be *little*, and you might hear utterances such as *little* dog, *little* flower, and *little* bug.

Since these 2-word utterances are not complete sentences, their meanings are determined by the context and the intonation the child uses, as in holophrases. For example, "Little ball?" spoken with the upward intonation of a question might mean, "Can Daddy get the little ball for me?" Of course this also gives you the opportunity to expand this utterance ("Do you want Daddy to get your little ball?") and interact with your child. This is a very exciting time for baby because he is now able to communicate his desires more and more effectively, and he is really learning the power of language. Before long he will be putting together three or more words and speaking in sentences.

Are there best ways to talk to my baby at this stage?

Yes. In fact, an appropriate way to talk to your baby will probably come naturally to you. When babies are learning language, parents typically use a type of language that used to be called "motherese." But since fathers, other caregivers, and even older children also use this style of language with toddlers, it is now called infant-directed speech (IDS) when talking to babies, and child-directed speech (CDS) when talking to toddlers.

This type of speech has a musical quality to its pitch and rhythm, pitch being slightly higher and rate slightly slower than normal speech. Sentences are short and simple ("Give me the ball" rather than "Please hand the ball to me") and there is some very limited use of "baby talk" ("ba-ba" for bottle, "din-din" for dinner). Key words are also emphasized for meaning. Parents using IDS and CDS are also very responsive to their child's utterances. Even when baby is babbling, Mom will respond as if she knows exactly what baby said. But remember that this type of speech is for babies – not for 4-year olds. That means it is for very young children who are just developing language skills, not for children about to enter kindergarten.

By the way, adults and older children also use CDS when speaking to animals. In fact, even toddlers use a type of CDS when talking to babies and animals. Have you noticed how you speak to your cat as if he could understand you better if you used a high pitched, simple sentence while smiling? "Where's the good kitty?" and "Are you the best kitty?" are normal questions to many cats, who immediately come over for a scratch under the chin.

Does it sometimes seem silly to use CDS with little ones? It shouldn't. It gives parents and babies a kind of communicative intimacy, and babies attend well to it, possibly because the pitch and rhythm easily activate the right hemisphere, which is slightly more developed in babies than is the left. Babies love "sing-songy" words and phrases, even when they don't understand the words. Prosody comes first; words come later.

Can I hurry my child's sentence development?

As was explained above, toddlers quickly progress from one- to two-word utterances, and there is a normal range of time for this to happen. Toddlers will learn sentence types when they are ready, even when parents try to teach them more complex sentences. In fact, when parents and caregivers "correct" what a child has said, they correct his truthfulness, not his grammar.

This is what usually occurs:

Annie: Gween fower.

Mom: (correcting the truthfulness of the sentence) No, Honey, that's not a green flower, it's a bush.

Annie: (looks puzzled, but listening)

Not this:

Annie: Gween fower.

Mom: (trying to correct syntax) Honey, say, "Look at the green flower."

Annie: Gween fower!

(It is as if the toddler doesn't hear the correction at all and is upset because Mom obviously didn't hear what she had to say.)

Toddlers learn to use sentences when they are ready, but they help themselves develop by constantly engaging in dialogs to practice their language skills. They often contribute two or three sentences at a time to conversations, unlike babies, who "do their own thing." Three-year-olds also want to understand, so they might ask for clarification by saying, "huh?" or looking confused. During this period they will also learn how to clarify when others are confused, generally by speaking louder or by speaking more clearly.

Your child is constantly experimenting with language at this age. You will hear him frequently overgeneralizing the morpheme "ed" for past tense and "s" for pluralization, coming out with sentences like "Daddy comed out with me" and "I see my foots." This demonstrates that your child's brain is really working to figure this all out. Soon he will be saying, "Daddy came out with me" and "I see my feet," but one has to learn a rule before knowing where to apply it. Although language is rule driven, there are, of course, many exceptions to the rules which also need to be learned. It takes time to crack the grammar code.

Who are the children who learn language well?

Researchers suggest that they are the children whose parents and caregivers do the following:

- ➢ Ask them questions
- ➢ Engage them in conversations
- ➢ Read to them often
- ➢ Expand their utterances

➢ Are good role models of language
➢ Show them how to be social and to get along with others
➢ Want to know what their children think about things and events
➢ Stay on their child's topic longer
➢ Try to understand their child's attempts at communication

They are also children who hear fewer commands from parents. That doesn't mean parents should not tell children what to do, but it should be a very small percentage of the language the child hears. "Turn down the TV," "Go out and play," and "Get over here" might at times be necessary, but these commands don't teach children *The Joy of Language*. Children should enjoy using language to interact with others, learning through language, following directions well, and being heard and respected.

You've noticed that the list above also includes reading to your child. Even before your baby understands much spoken language, read to her every day. A child held close on an adult's lap, listening to a story and being directed to pictures, is an experience that will lead your child to the love of books. What a wonderful way to be close to an adult, to learn new words and sentences, to memorize favorite phrases, and to appreciate the joy of written language! Then, when she is ready to use some of that language herself, she will start imitating words and phrases on her own.

Auntie Frieda: See the cow?

Ethan: Cow!

Auntie Frieda: Yes, the cow is eating grass. It says, "Moo"!

Ethan: Moo!

Auntie Frieda: That's right. The cow says "Moo"!

When will my child learn longer, more complicated types of sentences?

This takes a while. For young children it is much easier to comprehend language in a linear fashion – the subject of the sentence is doing something. "The dog is chasing the cat" means the dog is doing something. "The dog is chased by the cat" or "The dog knows the cat is chasing him" both mean the cat is doing the chasing, even though "dog" comes before "cat" in the sentence. Simple, linear sentences are easy to understand; other sentence structures are too difficult for very young children.

Between the ages of two and three, your child will have a tremendous growth spurt in sentence formation. You might, in fact, hear sentences containing 10 words or more, occasionally including the conjunctions *and* and *so*, uttered by your three-year-old. That's pretty amazing, knowing how complex syntax can be. You'll hear articles, prefixes and suffixes, irregular verbs, prepositions like *on* and *in*, contractions like *don't* and *can't*, and even some cause and effect relationships. ("Johnny is crying 'cause Tammy hit him") That doesn't mean your child will be ready to give speeches, but many three-year-olds are pretty verbal.

Three-year-olds often relate sequences of events, but usually without the appropriate use of "and." He might say, "At school we eat snacks. We play outside. We sing songs." It won't be for another year or so that he will say, "We eat snacks, play outside, and sing songs." This sentence formation involves the understanding that the pronoun "we" is understood in the last two sentences and that a string of related phrases require the "and" before the last one. This is a very sophisticated knowledge of our syntactic rule system that most children master before kindergarten.

97

All languages are rule driven, and some rules don't seem to make a lot of sense. For example, in many other languages, the adjectives come after the noun, which, when you think about it, makes much more sense than adjective placement in English. If the English noun is "house," when describing this house we might say "large, gray, dilapidated, hundred-year-old" before we even let the listener know that we're talking about a house. We have to hold pictures or concepts of these adjectives in our memory until we actually have an object to picture as having these attributes. Does that make sense? But we all learn the exact sequence of adjectives that come before a noun. (You wouldn't say "dilapidated, gray, large …") Could you explain the rule for this, though? Probably not. But many children unconsciously know it before 5 years of age.

Another language skill that is difficult for toddlers is learning to use pronouns that match the perspective of the speaker. When you say "my shorts" your toddler understands that meaning as the shorts that belong to Mom. He doesn't call all shorts "my shorts," but understands the difference between *my* and *your*, and *mine* and *yours*. In fact, the word *mine* becomes very important to the three-ear-old, especially when it comes to toys. Have you ever heard a toddler call Daddy's car "my car" because that's what Daddy calls it? When you take a toy away, though, you will most definitely hear, "Mine!"

Between two and three your child will also begin with the sometimes incessant use of the word *why*. Since it is difficult to formulate whole sentences that begin with *why*, and it's not necessary, this famous word of two-year-olds is usually uttered all by itself.

Mommy: Stay with Daddy while I go to Aunt Jenny's for a little while.

Jenny: Why?

Mommy: Because she wants to see me.

Jenny: Why?

Mommy: Because she has some errands for me to do for her.

Jenny: Why?

Mommy: Because she has a cold and doesn't want to go out.

Jenny: Why?

Mommy: Because she might get even sicker.

Jenny: Why?

Mommy: Because it's very cold out today. And that's it. Bye-bye. I'll be home soon.

Very soon your child will begin to ask "wh" questions other than "why" (*who, what, when, where,* and *how*). But it will be very difficult for him to concentrate on using the question inversion, changing the order of the noun and verb ("Where is Bobby?" rather than "Where Bobby is.") while focusing on these question starters.

Michael: Where Mommy is?

Dad: Where is Mommy? She's at the store.

Michael: When Mommy's coming home?

Dad: When is Mommy coming home? Pretty soon.

Toddlers also learn to use a kind of shorthand of language that we call "ellipsis," leaving out portions of conversations that are already understood by both parties. This shorthand makes our conversations so much more efficient. Teachers of young children often ask them to answer with a full sentence in order to teach children what a sentence is, but much of our daily language does not contain full sentences, nor should it. We do not have to mention everything we are communicating. Consider this interaction:

Grocer: Did you find everything okay?
Customer: Are you out of Brussels sprouts?
Grocer: They're over by the lettuce now.
Customer: Oh, thanks.

Now let's look at the same interaction without ellipsis:

Grocer: While you have been in this store today, were you able to find everything you were intending to buy?

Customer: I found everything I intended to buy except the Brussels sprouts. I went to the place in the produce section where I have found them in the past, but they were not in that place. Other similar items were there, though, so I thought you had already sold all the Brussels sprouts and had not yet received a new shipment of them.

Grocer: We do have Brussels sprouts and they are stocked on a shelf in produce. We moved them from the place where we previously stocked them and put them on the shelf next to the lettuce.

Customer: Thank you for the information about the new placement of the Brussels sprouts. I will now return to the produce section and will look for them in the place that you explained to me during this interaction.

The first conversation was much easier, wasn't it? Aren't you glad that so much is understood, and that we can use ellipsis?

Then, of course, there will always be the ambiguous sentences that even adults might not understand without being well aware of the context. A rather famous linguistic example is the sentence "The chicken is too hot to eat." If the speaker is in a very hot barnyard, she may be telling you that the chicken isn't eating because of the heat. If the speaker has just taken a chicken out of the oven, she is probably warning her family not to start eating it yet. The syntax is identical in each situation, but the meaning is very different. So besides learning to string words together, your toddler is also learning that you can't always depend on those strings of words.

As you become more aware of how we use language, you will begin to understand how much your child is learning about it and what an incredible skill he is developing. Listen to your own language, to how you and others are interacting in conversations, to how you are speaking to your child, and to the words, sentences and body language you and he are using every day. What can you expect him to understand and to say as his language develops? It is limitless.

How can I make sure my child will be prepared to understand and learn the language of school?

Reading, writing and spelling will be discussed in chapters 8 and 9, but you can begin by being aware of any speech or language difficulties your child might be demonstrating in articulation, vocabulary, grammar, or understanding.

Children with moderate to severe speech sound (articulation) disorders have scored significantly lower on morphological awareness measures as well as on phonemic awareness, word-level reading, and spelling tasks. These language awareness difficulties may result in difficulties acquiring literacy skills. Simple sound substitution difficulties (e.g., w/r or θ[th]/s) will most likely not affect literacy at all, but children with multiple articulation errors might have difficulties with phonemic awareness, resulting in difficulty in learning to read.

Children who do not have an internal "feel" for grammar are also likely to exhibit reading delays. Teachers often use strategies like miscue analysis (noting the errors a child makes during oral reading) and asking a child if what they just read "makes sense." Many children with language problems don't know whether it made sense. They are often so confused that confusion is normal for them; thus, they really don't know the difference between confusion and understanding – or what "makes sense." In fact, they will often tell the teacher that it doesn't make sense because they know that if it did make sense, the teacher wouldn't be asking them that question. Yes, kids pick up on "teacher cues" very quickly.

Once a child is in school, most of her language assignments are metalinguistic. That means that they require the child to think about language. When a teacher asks, "Does that sound right?" he is really asking the child to make a judgment about language. When your child is two or three, you don't expect him to think much about the words he is using; you're just happy that he is speaking well for a toddler. When he is in first grade, though, and learning to spell, he is expected to think about what word the sounds "m-a-n" make. "M-a-n? Does that sound like 'man'?" Now he's got to put on his metalinguistic cap to think about the sounds of his language. Is his language developed enough to allow him to reflect on it? This is where all your years of preparation are really going to pay off.

Much of what will be expected of your child in school is metalinguistic. It will require the foundation that you have built with your child in the preschool years. Think back to those years in school when you learned about articles, pronouns, nouns, verbs, adjectives, adverbs, clauses, etc. Your teachers did not talk about types of words, the "parts of speech," until you were already using them with relative ease. These were metalinguistic lessons – lessons that asked you to reflect upon your own language. Language acquisition comes first; learning about language comes later.

Will our family's dialect affect my child's learning?

All languages are dialects because they have specific regional and cultural vocabulary, grammar and pronunciation. In the United States, however, most teachers believe they have an obligation to teach what we call Standard American English, although there are also differences within the "standard." Some teachers call the language of school "school talk," or something similar. There is certainly nothing wrong with other forms of grammar, vocabulary and pronunciation – even other ways of writing (e.g., email and texting). But since texts, novels, articles, web sites, etc. are mostly written in Standard English, and teachers teach in Standard English, it is necessary for students to be able to understand this type of English and to be able to write adhering to these standards. By learning Standard English they are adding to their repertoire of language and languages. Cultural, geographic and family dialects and languages are very important because they connect us to others. But being able to speak in different ways with different people is a skill that will prove to be very useful. So speaking, writing and reading the "standard," in addition to speaking your family's dialect, will make academic learning easier and will support your child's success throughout life. This topic will be discussed further in Chapter 7: Dual Language Acquisition and Dialects.

SHARING THE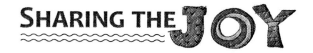

♥ Chat with your baby and toddler as if he understands everything you are saying so he hears many examples of sentences with different vocabulary and prosody.

♥ Always be a great role model for language – your child is learning language by listening to you.

♥ Join your child in pretend play and speak like the characters to encourage dialogue.

♥ Expand your child's utterances without telling her you are correcting her word pronunciation or grammar.

♥ Use a lot of self-talk, narrating what you are doing and thinking, as your child listens.

♥ Use parallel talk, narrating what your child is doing, while she plays, helps with chores, etc.

♥ Encourage talking by listening attentively and responding to her questions and comments.

♥ Give him time to figure out what to say – being rushed can be frustrating to him – and wait a few seconds for him to formulate his sentence.

♥ Use sentence completion when reading story books to your child: "Where is the bear? The bear is _(behind the tree)_."

♥ Play a game of morphemes with objects and actions: Say, "Here is an apple, and here are two _(apples)_." "Yesterday I hopped, but right now I am _(hopping)_," having your child fill in the missing word.

♥ Ask open-ended questions (not questions that can be answered by "yes" or "no") about an experience or what is happening in a story: "What did you do at the park with Daddy?"

♥ Look at ads in magazines with your child and ask, "What do you think she's saying?"

♥ Talk about past events and ask questions about what happened to practice past tense.

♥ Play "concentration" with picture cards in pairs to practice plurals: "I have two bicycles!"

♥ Cut out pictures from magazines and have your child describe each with short sentences so you can guess the picture he's holding.

♥ As a metalinguistic activity, count words in sentences by using your fingers, then have your child count the fingers.

♥ Look for prefixes and suffixes in words when reading with your preschooler – talk about how they change meaning (tie/untie, appear/disappear, run/running, beauty/beautiful).

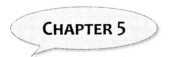

CHAPTER 5

Sounding Like Language: How Prosody Makes It All So Interesting

Spoken language has another extremely important element: prosody. This has been mentioned previously, but it also deserves a more in-depth discussion. Prosody, or the prosodic features of a language, is the pattern of stresses, pauses and intonation that makes the oral language interesting and adds a great amount of meaning to the utterance. It is both expressive and receptive. We use our vocal intonation to tell the listener what our words really mean, and we understand what people really mean by the way they say it. Prosody is an important characteristic of each language; besides pronunciation, it is what enables us to know what language someone is speaking even if we don't know one word of that language. Different cultures and languages use different prosody. It makes it all so interesting!

How does prosody change the meaning of sentences?

You can utter the same sentence with exactly the same words and mean entirely different things depending on the intonation and stress patterns you use. When we are joking, sarcastic, upset, frustrated or serious, we express it through the prosodic features of our speech. Can you imagine not being able to interpret people's feelings? Some children and adults can't, and this makes true communication very difficult.

Here is a little exercise to illustrate prosody. Read these sentences aloud, putting the emphasis on the words written in bold font. The implied messages are in parentheses.

1. **Do** you want coffee with dessert? (Have you changed your mind about not wanting coffee?)

2. Do **you** want coffee with dessert? (Everyone else does, do you?)

3. Do you **want** coffee with dessert? (Or are you still deciding?)

4. Do you want **coffee** with dessert? (Or would you rather have tea?)

5. Do you want coffee **with** dessert? (Or would you rather have it later?)

6. Do you want coffee with **dessert**? (Or would you rather have it with your meal?)

As you can see, the way we say each sentence adds as much of the meaning as the words themselves. Prosody is often the key to correct interpretation.

When do babies learn prosody?

Babies are exposed to the rhythmic patterns of the language they hear around them from birth. As soon as the third month of life, infants and mothers imitate each other's prosody. This is a very important period of language development – learning to control vocal tones to match those of parents and caregivers.

Babies' receptive language areas of the brain attend to prosodic features very early in life. A nine-month-old baby can even tell the difference between the language of her parents and a foreign language. A baby will turn her head toward someone speaking her own language rather than someone speaking a language with different prosodic features. Babies are great listeners. They hear utterances like, "WHEN should we GO to VIsit Aunt SAlly?" with stresses on specific syllables and, although she might not understand the words, she knows that it is her language and that it sounds familiar and interesting.

Prosodic stress, along with patterns of phonemes, is also important in enabling the infant to learn names of objects. He recognizes that this is probably a word because he hears it frequently, and it is often pronounced with a little more volume than other words (especially content words) in phrases and sentences. So he focuses on that word and recognizes it when he hears it again. As you can see, prosody plays a very important role in the learning of language.

When will my baby begin to use prosody?

Listen to your baby babbling – not using words, only uttering strings of sounds. If English is the language of the home, your baby is babbling in English. You can tell that she is because you can hear English prosody in the strings of sounds. It does not sound like Chinese or Swedish babbling.

The words and sentences are produced in the left hemisphere, but the right hemisphere contributes to the underlying meaning of each spoken sentence. Prosody is the first aspect of language that is acquired – long before baby's first words. Your baby is using prosody to communicate needs and to figure out what language is all about. Because of this, talking to your baby, reading stories, and singing songs are all necessary for language development. Songs and stories engage children with the prosodic features of rhythm and melodic patterns that boost brain capacity and improve language and memory. Isn't it easier for you to remember the words to songs if you sing the melody? It's easier for babies, too, to remember words and sentences when they can remember their rhythm.

Do mothers and fathers use different prosody with their babies?

Studies have found that mothers employ consistent prosodic cues when speaking to their young children, putting stress on important and new words. This is also a way to express emotion and to teach sentence structure when reading to the child. But infants and toddlers can also learn so much from fathers and other male adults reading to them and interacting with them using poems, songs, jingles and finger plays that immerse the child in a "man style" of speaking and caring. Sometimes men are reluctant, or think it is silly to use exaggerated prosody, gestures, and facial expressions with babies, but men are very receptive to learning this and love to watch their babies respond with such joy!

SHARING THE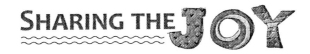

- ♥ Imitate your baby's cooing, and he will imitate many of your sounds.

- ♥ Read him bedtime stories that are comforting, using a relaxing tone of voice, even if he doesn't understand all the words or content.

- ♥ Use some exaggerated prosody when talking with your baby or toddler – she will find this fascinating and stimulating.

- ♥ Sing songs and jingles to get him used to listening for tone and rhythm.

- ♥ Ask questions of your baby, even if she can't respond, to model the prosody of questioning.

- ♥ When talking about objects, actions or people, use more stress for new vocabulary words.

- ♥ Reflect his feelings with facial expressions and intoned phrases.

- ♥ Play different kinds of music to her, some soft and gentle, some more lively, and "dance" with her to the rhythm.

- ♥ Read stories to your child using different voices for characters, and ask him to guess who is speaking now – good practice for tuning in to the ways different people speak.

- ♥ Have her imitate your prosody by saying short sentences (like "What are you doing?") with the emphasis on different words – also a great metalinguistic game because it illustrates individual words in sentences.

♥ Role play with your preschooler: Ask "How would you say that if you were sad? Angry? Afraid? Upset?"

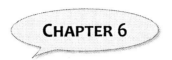

CHAPTER 6

Social Language: The Pragmatics of Communicating

The word "pragmatic" means dealing with specific problems in a logical way. We use our language for specific purposes, or to solve specific problems, like to ask for something, to compliment someone, to get someone's attention, to express anger, to think about the world, etc. These are examples of the pragmatic aspect of our speech and language. We are successful when we solve the problem – when we communicate what we intended.

All cultures have pragmatic rules, and most of the rules are what we call "social skills." We generally learn these rules through observation and practice, but don't be surprised if your child needs a little extra help with these social skills. Many children do. Since you are your child's pragmatic role model, here is what you need to know.

Are there many different ways to use language socially?

Absolutely. Social communication is the first language your baby will learn, because it is the first language she will need. But she will be communicating with you long before she begins to use words. Naturally, your baby has desires and needs. How will she get her needs met? First, of course, she will use non-verbal communication; later, she will express her needs with words, sentences, conversations and writing.

Think about what we need to know about appropriate social communication. Do we express ourselves with tact? Do we take turns in conversations? Do we give the listener just the right amount of details without going on and on and on? Do we clarify our ideas for the listener? Do we talk to ourselves when trying to solve a problem?

Few of us think about all the ways to be appropriate in social situations; it just comes naturally for most of us. We know how to act and what to say, and what not to say, in all types of settings. We all use language in a variety of ways every day.

Think about some of the things we do easily with language:

- Take turns during a conversation
- Use appropriate eye contact when speaking with someone
- Remain on topic until transitioning to a new topic
- Ask questions of a conversational partner for clarification
- Respond to a speaker's questions
- Make requests
- Speak loudly enough to be heard, but not too loudly
- Use appropriate formality or informality for the situation
- Tell stories in an organized way
- Give enough, but not too much, information during a conversation
- Stand close, but not too close, to a conversation partner
- Take cues from a conversation partner (non-verbal cues that say she is bored, confused, getting angry, etc.)
- Speak tactfully so as not to make others feel uncomfortable
- Use prosody, and usually facial expression, to indicate sarcasm
- Know when something is funny – have a good sense of humor
- Contribute to group discussions appropriately
- Argue and debate skillfully

- Speak the jargon of different groups
- Possibly switch dialects for different social/cultural groups
- Say the correct things for social rituals ("Happy birthday!")
- Understand others' points of view from listening to their words, watching their body language, and being aware of their intonation

Have you ever really thought about all the skills you have for maintaining social communication? Think about this as your child is learning to interact appropriately through language. He has so much to learn.

How do our brains "understand" social situations?

The pragmatics of language is mostly a function of the right hemisphere. The right hemisphere processes much information as a whole, sometimes called the "gestalt." The gestalt is the overall idea, the social setting, where bits and pieces of information fit, so that we can determine what they mean within that social situation. It informs us about the social context so we can use and interpret the melody and rhythm (musical qualities) of language, and can use and interpret visual information in that setting.

Think about what aspect of language is related to melody and rhythm. Prosodic features, of course. As was demonstrated above, you can say two sentences with exactly the same words but with different intonation patterns and they will have two entirely different meanings. These meanings must be interpreted by listening to the way they are spoken. The syntax, or sentence structure, is processed mainly in the left hemisphere; prosody is processed mainly in the right, where the underlying meaning is discovered.

Now think about what aspects of communication might be affected by your ability to interpret visual information. How about facial expressions and body language? Could we communicate as effectively if we didn't understand what others meant by different facial expressions and gestures? So much of what we say depends upon how we say it – our intonation, volume, emphasis, facial expressions, hand gestures, the way we sit or stand, and many other non-verbal messages.

As you can imagine, people with right hemisphere deficits might not be able to use prosody that reflects their feelings, and also might not be able to understand the real meaning of the utterances of others. This can significantly disrupt social skills. But luckily most adults and older children have the capacity to understand social contexts so they can act accordingly. Younger children, though, still need much modeling, teaching and coaching.

How do babies begin to learn social communication skills?

Baby's first cry is the beginning of his connection to others through vocal communication. Did you react to your newborn's cry? Of course you did. And you probably responded with some vocalizations of your own – something like, "Ooohh!" Newborn babies don't cry in order to communicate something, but very soon they learn that parents respond to their cries, and a meaningful connection begins.

Please don't believe "experts" (often family members) who suggest that you let the baby "cry it out" rather than picking him up or going to comfort the baby when he cries. Babies do not cry to make your life unbearable; they cry because they are in distress and they need to be attended to. When this is your baby's only way of communicating, it is important for him to be able to trust that you are listening. Your attention will not "spoil" him or increase his crying. In fact, researchers have shown that babies whose caregivers responded to their needs more often actually decreased crying at about eight or nine months. It may be that these babies feel that communicating their needs is effective, and they are more likely to be comforted by that feeling. They are also quicker to learn alternate means of communication: eye gaze, pointing and vocalizing. So attend to your baby's crying, knowing that the joy of conversation is not far away.

It will be a couple of months before your baby will be able to practice another important aspect of communication – eye contact. The vision of a newborn is extremely poor, approximately 20/200. In fact, even the vision of a 1-year-old is not totally clear. But making silly faces, holding a teddy bear in different positions where baby can find it, and hanging mobiles over her crib all prepare baby for eye contact. A 2-month-old might not see clearly; however, she can recognize faces of primary caregivers. So provide your baby with visual stimulation. The visual cortex, as other parts of the brain, needs interaction with the environment for proper development.

As your baby develops eye contact, she will also become fascinated by facial expressions. This is such an integral part of the way we communicate feelings. When you hold the baby so she can see your face, or when you lean over her crib and smile, she is studying one of the most important aspects of human communication. It is so exciting to see that your baby is captivated by your face, your voice, and even your walk. She is now watching and listening to everything you do and say. She is learning quickly to use all forms of communication with you, her greatest teacher.

What should I notice in my baby's pragmatic language development?

Notice your baby's body language, eye gaze, and facial expressions in reaction to things. Also notice his curiosity and interact with him around his interests so he will know that he is telling you his likes and dislikes. Before babies can talk, they can convey many messages nonverbally. *Rejection* is conveyed by a head shake of "no" or pulling back from something unwanted. Babies *request* things by pointing and vocalizing. They *comment* on things by showing them to adults, vocalizing and gazing. When they look at Mom or Dad and signal that they want to "discuss" something, they are happy when Mom or Dad names the object and comments on it. This not only teaches baby new vocabulary, but it also enables parents to see how pleased baby is when someone correctly interprets what he is trying to "say."

Within the first year, much of the communication intent is represented by body language. Hands up in the air means "Pick me up"; pointing to the bottle means "I want more milk"; turning the head away means "I don't want any more." Start to notice, in yourself and others, how much meaning is conveyed through body language: gestures, eye contact, body postures, facial expressions, amount of distance between the speaker and listener. Your baby notices, too.

How do toddlers learn to use language in socially appropriate ways?

They learn by watching and listening. Although we do teach our children "manners," nearly all of their social communication skills are learned from watching us. Just think of all the appropriate, and inappropriate, ways there are to use language and other behaviors in different situations. Just as we can't teach our children syntax (we can only model it and sometimes correct their grammar), we also can't teach them how to act and what to say in every social setting they might encounter throughout their lives.

Toddlers learn through daily experiences and daily routines, like getting dressed, eating breakfast, nap time, bath time, and visiting their favorite fast-food restaurant. These are perfect settings in which to practice "scripted" language for communication. Often when youngsters are put into a totally new situation they are too preoccupied with the experience to also practice language skills. But familiar situations allow for great practice with the kinds of questions, comments and vocabulary that are appropriate for the situation. For example, during bath time your toddler can comment about taking clothes off, testing the temperature of the water, playing with her rubber ducky, getting her hair washed, and being dried off to put on pajamas. Although at a new restaurant for Auntie Pat's birthday, she might just look around in amazement, too overwhelmed with the new situation to eat, or to even think about talking. Upon her third visit to that restaurant, however, she will be ready to learn.

How will social language develop once my child is talking?

The social use of language is expressed verbally almost as soon as baby learns her first word. "Hi" and "Bye-bye" are usually the first "social" words baby learns. They indicate a ritualistic politeness when first seeing someone or leaving them. In fact, parents often instruct baby to "Wave bye-bye," and then soon after to "Say bye-bye."

It is important to most of us to socialize our children not only so their actions and words will be acceptable, but also so we are not embarrassed by their behavior in public. Of course, it is inevitable that we will at times be embarrassed by our toddlers because we can't teach them what to say, and what *not* to say, in every situation. All parents experience some awkwardness when their toddler in the supermarket very loudly says something like, "Look at the lady with the funny hair!"

And sometimes parents are surprised by another important pragmatic event which occurs when a child is around two years of age – the beginning of a sense of humor. All of a sudden your child will begin to realize that she can experiment and play with oral language, and actually begin to make "jokes." She might call objects or people by the wrong name and then laugh. Or she might use funny words, as in "Debbie is a poo-poo." She might even make up her own funny words to interject into sentences, showing that she knows she is substituting words. Although 2-year-olds are still pretty metalinguistically unaware, you can see this skill beginning to emerge.

Is it difficult to learn to have a conversation?

Do you remember how you learned to have a conversation? Did anyone teach you? Do you now know how to have a conversation? Of course you do. But could you explain it to anyone else, step by step? Probably not. In fact, having a conversation is a very complex process with specific rules that most of us learned by observing, practicing, making errors, correcting ourselves, and practicing some more.

You've probably never considered how many discrete skills are needed just to have a conversation. Understanding facial expressions and body language, knowing when to interject your thoughts without being rude or overbearing, and knowing when you need to clarify or add details. These are all learned conversational skills. And, of course, before you even begin the conversation you need to know how much the listener knows about the topic. That will tell you whether you need to ask questions (e.g., "How do you know Jane?" or "Have you ever shopped at The Ugly Duckling?"). If you are friends with the person, most background information is implied, and doesn't have to be stated. There is really a whole choreography to having a conversation, and most of us can do it pretty well without ever having been formally taught.

You might never have thought much about eye contact during conversations, but can you imagine how important it is? For instance, did you realize that when you are the speaker in a conversation, it is polite to look off to the side every so often so as not to bombard the listener with both your voice and your gaze? When, on the other hand, you are the listener, it is perfectly appropriate to continue to maintain eye contact with the speaker. We learn these skills just from being in conversations with people who have these skills, and they are learned unconsciously.

Conversations require a lot of cooperation between and among participants. Participants must interject just the right amount of information – not too little or too much. We don't expect others to go on and on and on without a break when speaking with us. Then if someone wants to change the topic, some type of transitional statement is usually necessary. And even with all this complexity, your child will learn it all by observing and practicing, just as you did.

What other pragmatic skills should I be looking for?

Preschoolers are still learning to understand what people mean when they ask indirect questions. Most people in the U.S. learn that it is often more polite to request indirectly than to command someone to do something. If you would like your husband to pass you the beans at dinner, you might say, "Could you pass me the beans?" You would not expect him to reply,

"Yes," and then do nothing. Don't expect your toddler to understand this, though. It takes quite a few years to understand and to use this social strategy. If you tell your toddler, "This room is so messy," expecting her to put her toys away, you might be waiting a long time. "Please put your blocks in the box" will get you much better results. It's interesting to watch how this skill develops in your child. As with other pragmatic skills, children learn by watching and listening, then integrating that pattern into their repertoire of communication.

Another pragmatic skill that will develop over time is the ability to speak somewhat differently in different social situations. Most people would speak differently (somewhat more formally) when teaching a class than when speaking with a spouse or good friend. Much of this depends on how well we know our conversational partner. And, like it or not, people make value judgments about a person's language, and often decide whether a person is "worthwhile" (worth getting the job, worth being accepted into this college, worth doing business with, worth befriending, etc.) depending on the way they speak.

To sum up pragmatics: It's not what we say; it's how we say it.

How do fathers affect social development?

In studies conducted to investigate the impact of father-child relationships, it was found that fathers generally interact more with their children once they become toddlers and older, but not as much when they are babies. Of course, this differs greatly among families. Fathers seem to enjoy interacting with their children more when they can play, cooperate, follow some social rules, assert their own needs, make comments, and ask questions. Children's language skills seem to contribute to father-child interaction as much as father-child interaction contributes to children's language and social development.

Another interesting finding was that fathers who engaged in sensitive and positive play with their 4 ½ year old daughters had an impact on their child's social skills, even in the third grade. These children were regarded as being more cooperative, responsible, and self-confident.

Many fathers, of course, do engage in play with their babies and toddlers, and it has been demonstrated that this father-toddler toy play leads to better cognitive and social development. For that reason, it might be worthwhile to offer more training to fathers about how to have more play contact with their toddlers. There are, in fact, such courses offered throughout the country. They provide a wonderful opportunity for fathers to interact with their little ones in the company of other males. Mothers are always joining other moms for play group – now fathers can also have the support, camaraderie and fun!

How will my child's preschool work on her social skills and language pragmatics?

Being with other children with adult supervision will be giving your child many opportunities to practice social behavior and language. But many preschool children also need additional social skills training. Preschools usually offer this as a part of their curriculum, as well as focusing on social skills during group interactions and play time. Being able to share, to communicate thoughts and desires appropriately to peers, and to make requests politely are all learned skills that need to be taught. Many preschools use a social skills curriculum, and the teachers and caregivers focus on carryover of the skills throughout the day.

Another pragmatic language skill that can be taught and encouraged within a preschool setting is the use of sympathy and empathy. Besides being able to play well with others, it is also important for children to learn to use comforting words when appropriate. Children can be taught to respond to an emotional display of another child or adult, and also to judge whether the displayed distress is justified. In fact, they become quite good at this. The ability to imagine what other people are thinking or feeling is called "Theory of Mind," an important part of cognitive development. Studies have shown that preschoolers who exhibited this "emotion knowledge" were less likely to cry or behave aggressively in difficult situations. They were able to regulate their own emotions, seemed able to cope emotionally in kindergarten, and to be more socially accepted. Because of this, preschoolers benefit from teachers and parents instructing them on appropriate ways to express emotions and to respond to the emotions of others.

SHARING THE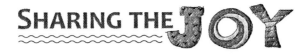

- ♥ Take crying seriously and soothe your baby – she is communicating a need.

- ♥ Try to figure out what your baby's various sounds mean.

- ♥ Use facial expressions to make your baby laugh and tune in to body language.

- ♥ Cuddle up during story time to make reading stories a comforting, enjoyable experience of listening attentively to a speaker.

- ♥ Use soothing gestures when he is upset – this will show him how to do the same with others.

- ♥ Show your toddler you are listening – nod your head, use good eye contact, make comments, ask questions.

- ♥ Don't overreact to exaggerated body language – he is most likely just practicing this form of communication.

- ♥ Always respond positively to cuddles – this will encourage interaction and engagement.

- ♥ Show pleasure and enthusiasm when your baby is trying to communicate with you.

- ♥ Verbalize her needs for her to show her she is already communicating, like "I know it's really hard to reach your Teddy, isn't it?"

- ♥ When talking to your infant, pause long enough for him to babble a response to you – to teach early conversational skills.

- ♥ Mirror your toddler's body language as a form of empathy – that you received her message and understand how she feels.

- ♥ Observe your child's facial expressions and body language so you can become a great interpreter of his moods and needs.

- ♥ Play with a toy telephone/cell phone having conversations with your toddler.

- ♥ Maintain rules, don't give in to tantrums, and use gestures for emphasis when saying "No" – showing that there are better ways to communicate frustration.

- ♥ Initiate pretend play with tea sets, dolls, toy kitchens and appliances, cans and boxes from the grocery store, etc.

- ♥ Use facial expressions that show you are listening to your toddler or preschooler.

- ♥ Use good eye contact with your child when you are communicating with each other.

- ♥ Demonstrate and talk about personal space. ("Oh, my goodness. I think you're standing too close to Jeremy to be using such a loud voice.")

- ♥ Praise caring gestures like putting an arm around another child to comfort him.

- ♥ Respect when your toddler needs time to just be quiet – thinking and problem solving are important aspects of pragmatics.

- ♥ Reprimand for negative touch (hitting, grabbing) – and encourage language use for communicating anger or frustration.

♥ Criticize the action, not the child, to show social appropriateness. (Don't say "You're a naughty girl," say, "Pulling Katie's hair is a naughty thing to do. That hurts.")

♥ Praise sociability when he talks to others.

♥ Encourage sharing and noticing the needs of others.

♥ Look for and use "teachable moments," frequently telling and showing your child how to act and what to say while experiencing a situation.

♥ Encourage your child to develop empathy and understanding by discussing people's motivations and emotions.

♥ Be very specific when praising your child, praising what she did ("That was very nice the way you said 'thank you' to Grandma") rather than for what she is ("You're so smart") – then she will know that she can become better and better.

♥ Make him aware of his body language. ("When you stand like that you look angry." "You look so happy smiling like that.")

♥ Limit access to her comfort objects to teach what is socially appropriate (like asking him not to take his blanket out into the yard).

♥ Encourage him to interact with others. ("Show Auntie Pat your new toy.")

♥ Get to know your child's communication style so you are not forcing her to be a "social butterfly" if that is not her inclination – she might feel more comfortable with one friend than in a group.

- ♥ Provide social opportunities like parent-toddler groups.

- ♥ Involve him in mealtime discussions – sitting, enjoying, and chatting with others.

- ♥ Keep dialogues going by asking for his opinion, commenting on his utterances and asking "wh" questions. ("Why …," "How …")

- ♥ Rehearse in advance what might happen in a specific social situation (e.g., going to a birthday party), what your child should say ("Happy Birthday, Judy!"), and tell her that she can find someone she knows to sit next to.

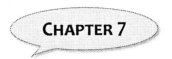

CHAPTER 7

Dual Language Acquisition and Dialects

Nowadays there are so many families moving from country to country that parents and teachers need to be knowledgeable about how to encourage children to speak more than one language. Young children are often expected to be fluent in one language at home and another language at school, sometimes serving as a translator for parents. Families have questions about the best ways to prepare their children to live within two or more languages, and frequently within more than one culture. Many parents, however, would like their children to speak more than one language for a variety of reasons. For instance, being bilingual, or multilingual, is often a sought-after qualification for employment in adulthood. Here are answers to some of the questions you might have when considering supporting your child's acquisition of more than one language.

Should I bring my child up to be bilingual if I can?

There are many advantages of being bilingual in addition to the most obvious – being able to communicate with many more people. There are also cognitive advantages to growing up bilingual. As has been explained already, one of the most important aspects of language development is metalinguistic awareness – the ability to think about language and to use it well. Since children who have the opportunity to interact in more than one language hear the differences in vocabulary and sentence structure, they have more of an awareness of the use of different sounds, words and sentences to symbolize meaning. You can imagine how helpful this becomes when asked to listen to phonemes and to learn new vocabulary in early elementary school. This awareness can even contribute to the ability to write for different audiences in higher grades.

There are also social and behavioral assets to being brought up bilingual. Studies have shown that bilingual children often outperform monolingual children on tests of abstract thinking and executive function, the ability to attend well and to focus on a goal. Pragmatically, many bilingual children also seem to have the ability to see the points of view of others and to take the perspective of people different from themselves. This may be because of their experiences with people of different cultures.

Exposure to another language early in life can also make it easier to learn additional languages later in life. While the brain is developing for language, the more the language areas are stimulated the stronger and more flexible they become. Learning more than one language in early childhood can encourage skills that will last a lifetime.

Can all children learn more than one language easily?

Most children can if they are exposed to each language at least 30% of the time. However, language disabled children have a much harder time acquiring a second language; they usually are not processing any language adequately enough to develop good linguistic skills. Children who are not reaching language milestones in their first language may be confused by the introduction of more than one language, just as they are confused by their first language. More about language disabilities will be discussed in Appendix A: Disabilities Affecting Speech and Language.

When children learn two languages early in life, do they retain the languages longer?

It depends on how often they are used. When a child learns more than one language simultaneously in a bilingual household, this process is actually language acquisition rather than language learning. Acquisition occurs when a child hears more than one language in many different naturally occurring situations throughout the day, and the language is used for communication. Acquisition is generally more long-term, but learning may be forgotten if not used in natural ways. When a child acquires language, she is unconscious of the process, just as she is while developing one language. Emphasis is on natural communication, not on the form of language. Because of acquisition, children and adults are able to tell what "sounds right," like "He runs every day" rather than "He run every day," without really having to think about it. Language learning, on the other hand, focuses on consciously learning the rules of a language. So children usually have less difficulty acquiring language, or languages, than learning a new language later. Whether a language is acquired or learned, however, it must be practiced and used in order to be sustained.

If I am not fluent in English myself, should I try to speak mostly English at home so my child will learn it?

Sometimes increased English usage at home is not really helpful, especially if parents are uncomfortable speaking English, and it may actually decrease the development of good language skills in the child's first language. Children need to hear fluent language in order to acquire it, so it is better for a child to acquire the form, content and use of one language well than not to be fluent in any language. Once a child's brain has acquired one language, he can learn literacy skills, for which language knowledge is essential.

In the earlier days of bilingual education, parents whose native language was not English were encouraged to use only English at home whenever possible because their children would be taught in English in school. But as a consequence, many parents who did not feel comfortable with English actually spoke less to their children so they wouldn't "hurt" them, and they never read to them because of not being able to read English. Finally it was discovered that learning any language well greatly improved learning and literacy in a second language. So please speak and read to your child in the language you know well, but also in a second language if you are able.

If we do not speak a second language at home, should my child take language classes before high school?

Some of the research on ESL is suggesting that the easiest time for a child to acquire a second language, if not from infancy, is ten to twelve years of age. But it is essentially never too late to learn another language. Younger children often have fun learning a new language, and they are not embarrassed by mispronouncing words or being grammatically incorrect. So starting young has its advantages. Then by ten or twelve, children's own language is structured enough so they can now develop a second language metalinguistically, so this is also an advantage. When students are older, however, they often take fewer risks. And, naturally, there are individual differences, skills and talents in language learning, as in all learning.

If we speak very little English at home and my child's preschool teaches in English, will my child learn English easily?

Preschoolers who do not speak English speak their home language, of course, when first in school. After they realize their home language is not working very well in that context, they usually become silent for a while. This gives them a chance to observe and to learn some words in English. Soon they will begin to try out these new words and phrases, using a combination of English and their home language. If they are in a supportive and friendly environment, teachers and other children will encourage them to speak and interact with ease. Preschool is a great place to learn and practice a new language.

The motivation to play with other children also accelerates the learning process. English-speaking children are generally very accepting of the language differences, and they just overlook errors in English. As long as the non-English speaking child is learning the social norms of the group, interacting and behaving appropriately, it is easy to maintain membership within play groups. Children find many ways to communicate – with words, gestures, pointing, sharing, and just having fun together.

Preschoolers generally take more risks using their new language during routine activities, like circle time when they discuss the weather and the activities of the day, recite rhymes and days of the week, and identify shapes and colors. Repetition, labeling, and singing build confidence in the new language in an enjoyable way. If the teacher is teaching something new to the whole group, however, it is more likely for the student to observe and to participate non-verbally.

If your child attends a preschool where some of the staff speaks his native language, he is, of course, at an advantage. Children who interact with preschool teachers in their first language are quicker to develop more complex sentences in their second language. Non-English speaking children in English-only preschools usually do not have the opportunity to learn English by having teachers point out cognates, words that are similar in both languages (like *market* and *mercado*). It is also advantageous, if possible, to leave about a half hour each day for instruction in the child's home language. Some pre-schools do provide this instruction for non-English speakers.

A preschool teacher who speaks the child's native language can easily provide a non-threatening environment for a non-English speaking child. For example, if a child is Spanish speaking, the teacher can use some Spanish words, provide children's books in Spanish, label items in the room in both Spanish and English, use both Spanish and English words while reading stories, play Spanish CDs, and play videos in which characters speak both Spanish and English. She can also model a nurturing relationship with the Spanish speaking child so other children will want to interact with him by playing and talking. And this has the additional benefit, of course, of exposing English speaking children to another language.

If my child speaks very little English, how will she understand the books read by her preschool teachers?

Studies have shown that rich explanations during story reading in the child's new language greatly accelerate the learning of that language. Even if the child has very little knowledge of the second language, when teachers take the time to explain English words to her in English, her vocabulary and understanding of English increases. Storybooks, especially ones with a lot of pictures, are a wonderful means of teaching new words – not just commonly used words, but also words that teach concepts in science, mathematics, other cultures, and a variety of experiences not found in everyday life.

Why are children who learn a second language able to master the accent of that language better than adult learners?

The reasons may be a combination of physiological, psychological and cognitive factors. It is possible that the brain acquires all aspects of language easier before there is specialization in the brain, so young children's brains acquire the sounds of more than one language more naturally. Adults also have a tendency to analyze new ways of doing things because of their later stage of cognitive development. This analysis might inhibit an immersion process. Also, since adults are usually more self-conscious than children, they may be more reluctant to try out "being" a Spanish, English or French speaker.

If my child is raised with a dialect of English, like African-American dialect or Chicano English, will that affect his success in school?

It might. Most teachers speak and teach in a standard American dialect, and they expect that their students will understand them – their vocabulary, grammar, meaning, intent, directions and explanations. When the form of school language is different from the form of home language, children have to become essentially bi-dialectical in order to flow easily from one way of communicating to another.

Sometimes teachers don't understand the significance of students using different words, sounds and grammar of various dialects because they perceive it as all English (or whatever is the standard language of the country). Some children who speak only a non-standard dialect are at a great disadvantage for classroom learning. When the way a child communicates, including the social uses of language (e.g. requesting information, being imaginative, being entertaining, etc.) is different from school expectations, the child's teacher might perceive difficulties with the child's learning or behavior, or both.

Trouble can also arise when teachers just expect students to know the difference between dialects. Since we don't really "teach" language, teachers often ask children, "Does that sound right?" expecting them automatically to know the form of standard American grammar. In fact, children who are raised in bilingual households sometimes have an easier time of deciding whether a sentence illustrates "good" English because they have more of a conscious knowledge (metalinguistic awareness) of language differences. Children who are raised with a non-standard dialect are generally introduced to Standard English by watching TV and movies, and playing videos, all passive experiences. They don't have opportunities to practice the standard form until they are in school, and then they are just expected to know it. This often becomes an obstacle to learning, and can greatly reduce reading comprehension.

To confuse the issue even more, many children who speak a certain dialect are taught in preschool by adults who speak another non-standard dialect. An African-American child may be cared for by an adult with a Latino-based dialect, and may, in fact, be understanding very little of what is being said in that preschool. It is important for parents to be aware of the differences between the home dialect and the dialects of their child's teachers. Living with dialect differences is certainly not unique to the United States, so parents throughout the world must understand the importance of their children knowing the language and dialect of the education system. As was stated in Chapter 4: Using Sentences, dialects are very important in connecting us to others, but being able to switch dialects is also a very valuable skill.

SHARING THE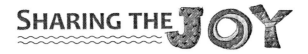

♥ Have one parent usually speak in one language and the other parent in the second language, if possible. (Research has shown that this strategy works well.)

♥ After asking a question, leave enough response time for your child to formulate the answer in the same language.

♥ Use a lot of prosody, gestures, body language and good facial expression in both languages.

♥ Encourage and be enthusiastic about attempts at speaking in each language.

♥ Arrange play dates with children who speak one or the other of your languages.

♥ Be consistent, expecting that your child will use and become fluent in both languages.

♥ Provide books, videos and music in each language.

♥ Use some household items that illustrate each language: placemats, posters, toys, plates, etc.

♥ Point out cognates – words that are similar in both languages.

♥ With older preschoolers, label items in the house in both languages.

♥ Read and use "Sharing the Joy" activities throughout this book, and share the joy in both languages!

PART 2:

Learning With Language

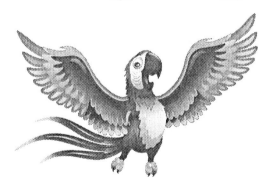

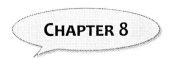

CHAPTER 8

Reading:
Figuring Out the Code

D o you remember how you learned to read? Was it so easy that you seemed to be born to read? Or would you rather not be reminded of the years of struggle to succeed at something that other kids had no problem with?

Although most children can become readers with the help of skilled teachers, you, of course, want your child to acquire the language and pre-reading skills necessary for literacy to come easily. Knowing about the process of reading and how it is affected by all aspects of language development will equip you to provide the necessary experiences for your child to become a reader – and to learn to love reading for a lifetime.

Is there a section of the brain specifically for reading?

Many areas of the brain are used for reading: parts of the temporal lobe, frontal lobe, occipital lobe, and other areas that connect pathways. But since brains have not changed much during the 5000 years since people have been reading, there is no "reading" area of the brain. Many of the world's languages, in fact, have no written form, although all societies have a combination of oral and gestural communication. Some researchers believe that this is because reading and writing are not natural processes for the brain in the way that oral or signed language is.

Reading is a fairly recent activity for brains, which are structured well for human language, but not for human reading. Reading involves brain circuitry that was actually evolved for other purposes. Still, most children can be taught to read. It is not surprising, though, that some have great difficulty convincing their brains that reading is normal. Some children have great difficulty with learning to read. This is often referred to as dyslexia. But, since there is not one specific portion of the brain which specializes in reading, dyslexia, or other learning disabilities, is not linked to exactly the same part of the brain in every individual. Reading with understanding requires processes from many areas of the brain. It is, like speaking, a much more complex activity than most of us realize when we do it so easily.

Can I teach my baby to read?

No. Babies can't read. As was stated above, reading is a complex process, and it is cognitively demanding. Babies do not have the cognitive skills to actually read, and there is no indication that holding flash cards up for your baby will accelerate her ability to read. Babies can be trained to clap their hands when they see the word CLAP on a card, and it's great to have the attention of a parent while playing this kind of game together, as long as it's fun and does not include the use of video (later about this in Chapter 11: Learning With TV and Other Media). Babies do not have the phonemic awareness, knowledge of the alphabet, vocabulary or sentence structure to actually read. It is entirely possible, though, that parents who use such programs also spend a lot of time playing with and talking with their babies – and that is the best indicator of a child's success in language learning, the necessary prerequisite to reading.

What pre-reading skills should I focus on?

All language skills are important for preparing your child to learn to read and to become a lifelong reader. As you already know, when babies hear interesting language and get an opportunity to interact linguistically with others, they develop better vocabularies, grammar, and other linguistic and cognitive skills. These skills then support their efforts in becoming good readers and writers. When children become better readers, they learn more vocabulary from books. They also become acquainted with various sentence structures which they can use in their oral language and writing. It is a cycle that is begun in infancy and continues for the rest of an individual's life: language → reading → language → reading. Parents and caregivers who give children a great foundation in language are empowering them to learn and to communicate well for life.

Pre-reading skills also include book knowledge: knowing how we use books. By the time your child is in kindergarten she should be able to choose a familiar book, "read" the title, hold it right side up, open it to the first page, "read" it from memory (tell the story in sequence by referring to the pictures), point to words, turn each page after "reading" it, and indicate the end of the book at the correct point.

Since children notice all ways that written language is used in their environment, it is also important to model using reading and writing in different ways each day. Parents can write notes to each other, use sticky notes to remember things, make grocery lists, send email, type computer searches, compose Word documents and print them out. When there are so many instances of adults and older siblings writing and typing, children enter school already motivated to learn how to do this. Pencils, markers, keyboards and pens are tools that your child will be excited to use – just like Mom, Dad, sister and brother.

When should I begin reading to my baby?

Although it may it may seem silly to read to infants when they don't understand the words or stories, it has, in fact, been shown that reading to infants, even before 6 months of age, can have a very positive impact on their language development and listening skills, and their eventual success in reading. So read to your baby as often as possible. It would also be worth your while to highly encourage your baby's caregiver to read to him daily.

Research has shown that children's development of vocabulary, auditory attention and listening comprehension, all very important in learning to read, are related to early exposure to books read with the child at home. As has been explained, it is not only words that are important, but also the intonation patterns of language – the prosody. Parents who read to their infants from birth exaggerate the prosodic qualities of the language, as they would with poetry. The prosody of expressive reading aloud is rich in melody and rhythm, which creates an affective connection between parent and child, a feeling of pleasure. The more the child experiences being read to, the greater will be the memory associated with feelings of pleasure. What a wonderful motivator to begin reading!

When your child is a toddler, you can have her "read" a book with you long before she can actually read any words on a page. Since this is such a pleasurable activity, "reading" picture books together can greatly enhance language and literacy. When looking at picture books together, ask her to "read" to you by telling you the story. She can point to the pictures that illustrate the story while you actively listen and ask her questions. You might ask, "Who is this?" "Why did she come?" "Tell me more about Sally." It's an easy and enjoyable way to encourage your child to practice many language skills: articulation, vocabulary, sentences, prosody and facial expression.

Should I focus on phonics when my child is very young?

It is unusual for very young children to be able to understand phonics, the relationship between letters and sounds, and how to blend them to make words. That is a cognitive skill that generally doesn't begin until about 6 years of age. It is important, however, to prepare your child by focusing on the sounds in words so that when phonics is introduced, the sounds will already seem familiar.

Parents and caregivers should focus on two types of auditory skills that are very important to learn before the teaching of phonics: phonological awareness and phonemic awareness. These are both components of good reading instruction, and they are explained below. Many studies have shown that the development of phonological and phonemic awareness, along with vocabulary, greatly affect the success of learning to read and write.

There are many different reading systems and programs that teachers use, and some work better than others for individual children. Most current reading programs do use a phonics-based approach, or one that at least includes phonics, so be sure to focus on the sounds in words with your toddler and preschooler.

Should I talk to my child more about language and reading?

Absolutely. If you want your child to learn to read more easily, here is the secret: focus on *metalinguistic awareness* from the time your child begins to talk. Metalinguistic awareness is the awareness and understanding that oral language is made up of sounds, sound sequences and words, and that language is a tool that can be used for a variety of purposes. It is the awareness that language can be observed and manipulated on a very conscious level. You can do this every day, many times a day, without taking any extra time at all from any activity or any task. You only have to be in the same room as your child.

145

Very young children do not yet have metalinguistic awareness, which develops with cognition, but you can encourage
this skill very early so that it will come easily when your child
is ready. A two-year-old will be able to express himself with
words, but he will not be able to really think about those words.
They just come naturally as he thinks of things he wants you to
know. Three- and four-year-olds, though, do begin to exhibit
some metalinguistic awareness. For instance, they might know
the difference between a picture, a written word, and a letter of
the alphabet, but they may still have difficulty counting words
in a sentence. It is not until about age six that a child begins to
understand that one can actually talk about language and not
just *use* it.

Some children who have difficulty in pre-reading activities in school are suspected of having auditory discrimination
problems, the inability to hear the differences between sounds
in words (like *pig-big*). If we think about metalinguistics,
though, we will discover that this might not be the case. If you
ask your child to turn his back to you and then to say "cat, bat,
rat," and he says it, he has obviously heard the differences. If,
however, you ask him if "cat" and "bat" sound the same and
he says "yes," that might mean he doesn't understand what
you're asking him, not that he doesn't hear differences. They
do sound the same in that they rhyme. He might also not be
able to tell you if they begin with the same sound because he
is not yet at that level metalinguistically. Or if he says they
are not the same, you don't know if he means they begin with
different sounds or they have different meanings. "Same" can
mean many things. Parents and teachers need to see tasks from
a child's perspective, which includes different levels of metalinguistic awareness.

Let's look at a third grade girl named Gina as an illustration
of metalinguistic ability. When Gina was given a test of meta-

linguistic awareness, a number of interesting things emerged. One subtest instructed Gina to determine whether an oral sentence was grammatically correct. She told the examiner that many of the ungrammatical sentences were correct. After scoring the test, however, the examiner read the same sentences aloud to her again. She asked Gina to imitate the sentences. She "imitated" each by correcting the grammar. If the examiner said, "The boys were *play* ball," Gina would say, "The boys were *playing* ball." Gina was repairing the sentences without even knowing that she was doing so. It was an unconscious process, but it is just this unconscious process, this lack of metalinguistic awareness, that is often the culprit that leads to academic failure.

Consciousness about sounds, words and sentences is the key. Talk with your child about what words sound like, what other word you might use to describe something, how to use different sentences (paraphrasing) to express an idea, and even different ways to emphasize words you are using. Be fascinated with language and your child will become a language expert.

What will my child be learning in reading instruction in school?

Good reading programs include the teaching of **phonemic and phonological awareness, phonics, fluency of reading, vocabulary** and **comprehension**.

Phonemic Awareness: This is the conscious awareness of the sounds of a language and the ability to manipulate those sounds – as in rhyming, blending phonemes and counting phonemes in words. Phonemic awareness is an auditory prerequisite of phonics. If your child has good phonemic awareness, she should be able to understand

and enjoy the following before she is expected to begin reading in the first grade:

- Rhyming – Twinkle twinkle little star, how I wonder what you are …
- Alliteration – Peter Piper picked a peck of pickled peppers
- Onset/rime – Separating the initial phoneme or phoneme cluster from the rest of the word (k – at)
- Beginning sounds – cake begins like Karen
- Ending sounds – car ends like star
- Phoneme addition – Add /k/ to at and get cat
- Phoneme synthesis – blending phonemes to make a word (/b/+/u/+/t/) = boot)
- Phoneme omission – Say cat without the /k/
- Phoneme substitution – If you take away the /g/ sound in goose and put in the /m/ sound at the beginning, what word to you have? (moose)
- Phoneme shifting to make new words – stop/tops
- Syllable omission – Say baseball, then say it without saying ball (base)

Phonological Awareness: This is the awareness of all levels of the phonemic system including phonemes, words, syllables, sentences and onset – rime. Phonemic awareness is part of phonological awareness. A child with phonological awareness knows what a word is, can count the number of words in a sentence, can clap out syllables, and so forth.

Some children have difficulty perceiving and remembering phonological information when processing written or oral language. Students with such phonological deficits have difficulty with phonics, reading, writing and spelling. They may also have articulation difficulties. Clarity of articulation does make phonemic awareness easier because children who cannot pronounce words correctly cannot play with sounds, which is one activity that leads to phonemic awareness. A few common errors will probably not interfere with learning to read, but multiple articulation errors probably will. Preschool children with speech and/or language disorders have responded positively to phonological awareness intervention, though this intervention may not be the only training a child needs in order to become a successful reader.

Phonics: Phonics is the use of phoneme/grapheme (sound/letter) relationships and the blending of sounds represented by letters to form words. It is the understanding that letters represent sounds and that we can blend these sounds into words, some with "regular" spellings and some with "irregular" spellings. Young readers should be able to "sound out" words and analyze similarities and differences in words.

Fluency: Fluency is the automaticity of reading, or reading without conscious effort. A child who reads fluently doesn't need to stop to sound out words and doesn't skip or substitute words when reading.

Reading fluency is necessary in order for the reader to comprehend meaning without expending energy in figuring out the words. One should be able to immediately gain meaning from the written words, sentences and paragraphs. Otherwise reading becomes a puzzle to figure out. But the puzzle is never really solved because the purpose of the letters and words is comprehension, which doesn't happen in the words, but in what we think about while reading. So you can see how important it is to be a fluent reader.

Vocabulary: A person's vocabulary is his understanding of word meanings (receptive) and the use of words to intend those meanings (expressive). Reading comprehension certainly depends on one's understanding of words, but it must be noted that this is only one requirement for reading comprehension (see below). For more information about vocabulary, please refer to Chapter 3: Learning New Words (Vocabulary) and Meaning.

Comprehension: Reading comprehension is the interaction of the reader with the text that allows the reader to construct meaning from what he is reading. Good readers interact with text: they question, make inferences, predict outcomes, and relate the ideas to their own lives.

Comprehension is dependent upon phonological and phonemic awareness, alphabetic knowledge, reading fluency, vocabulary, prior knowledge (including social knowledge), ease of processing sentence structures (syntax and morphemes), and interest in the subject. Reading comprehension is not just the understanding of individual words; it is the understanding of phrases, sentences and ideas expressed by the author and interpreted by the reader.

If you read other books and articles about the development of literacy skills, you might come across the term *Matthew Effect*. There is a passage in The Gospel of Matthew that refers to the rich getting richer and the poor getting poorer. What does this have to do with reading? It means that children who are read to, and who read a lot themselves, become better readers. They develop the vocabulary and other skills necessary to read fluently and to comprehend what they are reading. The more they practice, the better they become. But those children who are "poor" in their exposure to books become "poorer," or further and further behind their peers in reading and in school subjects that require reading for learning.

As you can see, acquiring a great vocabulary, being read to, and eventually reading a lot all contribute to becoming a life-long reader. Think about this: A typical first grader reads about 100 words and has a spoken vocabulary of about 6000 words; fourth graders recognize about 3000 words at a glance; fifteen-year-olds should recognize about 100,000 words quickly and read more than 200 words per minute. And it all begins with **phonemic and phonological awareness, phonics, fluency, and vocabulary**, leading to real **comprehension**.

What other skills are needed for reading comprehension?

Reading comprehension is, of course, the understanding of what we read. But there are so many details, words, and concepts both stated and implied in what we read that it is a much more complex task than just "understanding." Reading comprehension includes all of these skills, and more:

- Understanding the purpose for this specific reading
- Predicting outcomes
- Making inferences
- Understanding the main idea
- Visualizing characters, settings, and events
- Understanding the sequencing (beginning, middle, end) of a story
- Discovering cause and effect relationships
- Understanding plot development
- Knowing the author's purpose
- Understanding idioms, ambiguities and figurative language

- Understanding motives of characters
- Differentiating between fact and opinion
- Being able to interpret emotions
- Understanding the moral of the story

Many students are successful in reading through the second grade, because reading is more or less formulaic – sounding out and recognizing words, and predicting words within sentences. But in third and fourth grade, many children seem to develop learning problems that were not previously detected. Now they are expected to use their reading in a different way; they are expected to read to learn rather than to learn to read. At this point they get further and further behind in academics because of the new demands of their reading materials. Children who have learned to read first and second grade books don't necessarily have the skills listed above for more in-depth comprehension. This situation is much less likely to occur, however, when a child has a solid foundation in the important six aspects of language: phonology, morphology, syntax, semantics, pragmatics and metalinguistics. This foundation of language skills becomes the foundation for academic success.

If my child can tell me what she has read, doesn't that mean she understands?

Not necessarily. There is quite a difference between understanding and remembering. You most likely remember a lot of things that you don't understand. You might remember mathematical formulas without having an understanding of the derivation of the formulas and without knowing how to apply them. You have probably memorized poems in school, but that doesn't mean you really understood them.

The reading process needs to include **metacomprehension**, the ability to know whether you are comprehending or not. A reader must mentally interact with the message. It must mean something to him. Parents and preschool teachers can, and should, model this process for children. You might say, "I wonder what he meant when he told her she could do anything. Maybe he wanted her to try to ride the bike! Let's find out if we're right." This type of thinking out loud will show your child that reading is an active process of reasoning and reflecting.

Do you remember Gina, the student with poor metalinguistic skills? Well, Gina was also having reading comprehension problems. She had a good memory for details, though. After reading a story she could tell you every character's name, what they had done, and even what they had said. She had significant comprehension problems, though. But Gina had devised a system of fooling her teacher so the teacher didn't know how much trouble Gina was really having.

Gina's teacher would ask questions during reading group to check students' understanding. When she asked Gina, Gina's answers were far from the expected response. Since Gina was such a nice girl – fun-loving, helpful, good-natured – the teacher would ask Gina the question in different ways until Gina would finally come up with the right answer. Although there's nothing wrong with asking questions in different ways to help a child discover the answer to a problem, a teacher must be aware that this is what she's doing. She must discover how a child is thinking by listening to *every* answer. Parents need to do this, too. Can your child remember the slightest detail and yet be unaware of the messages implied in the story? Really listen to what your child says about the story – ask questions and listen to his first answers.

Don't children know when they don't understand?

Not always. Children often don't know what understanding means – they don't know the difference between understanding and confusion. When you or a teacher asks your child if he understands, and he says he does, it is somewhat difficult to be sure that he actually understands. Children often say they understand because they know that's what the adult wants to hear, and in school it often saves embarrassment or extra work for the child.

One cause of this confusion might be an effect of watching a lot of television. Whatever is happening on TV will continue to happen whether one understands it or not. Without a parent or other adult discussing the program with his child, many children never really know whether they understand the information, the plot or the implications. They focus on the action, the colors, the funny characters, or anything else they find interesting without understanding the gist of the program at all.

Because of this, many children don't make the connection between reading and making sense. They seem to see reading as a different process from thinking; they don't understand that reading *is* thinking. What we read needs to be related to what we know, to cause and effect relationships, to how the information can be used, to what might happen next, and so forth. You have to help your child make those connections right from the beginning so he will really know how different understanding feels from confusion.

What experiences will my child need for good reading comprehension?

Much has been written about the importance of children having good background knowledge, and many teachers are concerned about their students not having the experiences needed to understand what they are reading. Lack of physical familiarity with things your child is learning about, though, does not keep her from learning about people, cultures, nature, emotions, and anything else that can be discovered while reading.

Haven't you learned about other planets even though you've never visited one? Similarly, your child can learn about Koala bears even though she's only seen them on television. Taking trips, visiting museums, and going to fancy restaurants are certainly all occasions for learning, but it is wrong to expect less of children who don't have a wealth of worldly experiences. Children can learn from books, pictures, films, discussions, and social interactions as well as you can learn about Mount Everest without ever having climbed it.

In fact, even children who have a wealth of experiences don't necessarily learn from those experiences. We often have to lead them consciously through those experiences to ensure that they learn from them because many kids aren't used to doing that. Their attention is elsewhere – on whether it's time for lunch, on the discomfort of their new shoes, on negative emotions, on looking for places to run around, etc. We usually need to lead kids consciously to understanding. But we can do that if we all become teachers and role models for the excitement of learning – wherever we are.

SHARING THE 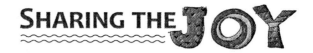 JOY

- ♥ When you read to your infant, be in a quiet, relaxed environment and hold him close to make this always pleasurable.

- ♥ If there are other siblings, frequently include them for story time.

- ♥ When reading nursery rhymes, use somewhat exaggerated prosody and a slightly louder voice on the rhyming words.

- ♥ Let your infant play with books made of cloth, cardboard or plastic, and even old magazines.

- ♥ Use different voices for different characters in the story.

- ♥ Act out some words with your voice. For example, for the word "snarl" you can actually snarl the word.

- ♥ Read your toddler's favorite story over and over again. Usually let him choose the story.

- ♥ Mealtime is a great time to focus on reading food labels. Do this for a few minutes (not through the whole meal).

- ♥ Have fun rhyming words with your food: toast, most, coast, boast, ghost!

- ♥ Point out syllables in the names of items and actions during household chores like setting the table, doing the laundry and making the beds. You can clap, step, or swing arms in rhythm to syllables (laun-dry, soap, T-shirt, un-der-wear, soft-en-er).

Start to share this JOY with your toddler, and especially with your preschooler:

- ♥ Use descriptive language, synonyms and explanations of words while reading to your child.

- ♥ Draw attention to rhyming words and, if he can, ask him to pick out the rhyming words himself.

- ♥ Clap out the words in a sentence with your child, then count the number of words together.

- ♥ Clap out the number of syllables in a word (one word at a time) while reading with your child.

- ♥ Count the letters in a word with your child.

- ♥ Leave off the last word of a sentence, but tell the child it rhymes with _____, and let her fill in the word.

- ♥ Point out words that have the same beginning sound.

- ♥ Ask "Wh" questions (Why, Where, When, Who, What, How) throughout the reading. Repeat your child's response and expand on it.

- ♥ Read books with your child that have a problem or solution. "What do you think he's going to do?" This teaches cause and effect, prediction, and making inferences.

- ♥ Prompt your child to "tell me more" or otherwise to clarify her answers.

- ♥ When reading to your child, stop and ask her to describe to you what she sees in her mind. "What do you think Jennie looks like?" or "What other people do you think might be there?" Good readers visualize what they are reading.

♥ Have your child fill in some oral "blanks," like "When Sally knocked on the door she was very _____."

♥ Listen to your child's answers to your questions and sometimes use them as conversation starters.

♥ Ask your child to predict "What might happen next?" or "How do you think the story will end?"

♥ Ask your child questions about the sequence of events: "What happened **first**?" "What was the **second** thing he did?" "What did she do **next**?"

♥ Connect the events or characters in the story with other stories you have read.

♥ Ask your child what the story was about (summarizing) after the book is finished.

♥ Explain words in the story that your child might not know and ask him to repeat the word.

♥ If you are reading a storybook with only a few sentences on each page, write a word on a card and ask your child to find that word on the page.

♥ Label parts of the book with your child and talk about each part: title ("What do you think the book is going to be about?"), author ("This is the person who wrote the book and thought up the story"), illustrator, photographer, etc.

♥ Ask your child to show you with her finger how you will be reading the book (left to right, top to bottom).

♥ After reading the story for understanding and enjoyment with your 4- or 5-year-old, go back over the story and make a game out of these activities:

- "Let's count the words in this sentence!"
- "Let's find the word _____!"
- "What is the first sound in _____?"
- "Let's listen for all the sounds in this word!"
- "What would this word, 'cat,' be if it started with a /m/?"
- "Here is the word 'mouse.' Which of these words doesn't begin the same as 'mouse'? Me. Mommy. Milk. Kitty."
- "What do you think this word is? b – e – d?"

♥ Show your child the similarities between speech sounds and visual letter patterns in words – show her how the "ch," "sh," and "th" make single sounds even though they are two letters.

♥ Use visual aids (like colored blocks) to illustrate sound blending: one color should represent each sound in a word. For example, say the word "cup." Put a green block, a red block and a yellow block in a row on the table. Touch the green block as you say the sound of "k," the red as you say the sound "uh," and the yellow as you say the sound of "p." Then say the word "pup" and change the green block to a yellow one (because the first sound is now different). Now there will be two yellow blocks, showing the word begins and ends the same.

♥ Model metacomprehension by asking yourself questions out loud for your child to hear. ("I wonder if he'll eat the apple. He said he was hungry, didn't he?) It will get him used to listening for meaning.

♥ Try to have your child follow along with her finger as you read aloud. Little by little have her quietly join you in reading.

♥ Use cloze procedure as you're reading with your child. While you're reading a story aloud that your child has heard many times, point to a major (noun, verb or adjective) word without saying it. See if the child can tell you what that word is. (Example: The next day in the forest they saw the same big _____.)

♥ Do not simplify vocabulary for your child. He should be learning new, more sophisticated vocabulary every day. Read the new word, define it, and use it in another familiar context. For example, "the ants were very *industrious* – they worked very hard. You are very *industrious* when you build with your Legos."

♥ Help your child pronounce difficult or long words. Have him imitate you syllable by syllable. Exaggerate the pronunciation and make it fun!

♥ Write labels on objects around the house: door, chair, floor, wall, table, etc.

♥ Read some informational books with your child, not just story books. Toddlers and preschoolers are interested in books about animals, insects, nature, the beach, and many other topics. Informational books also provide higher level vocabulary, like *antenna* and *magnetic*. These are words you can also use later, as when looking at insects or experimenting with magnets.

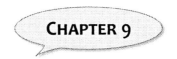

CHAPTER 9

Writing and Spelling

English, and many other languages, have a written form that is generally based upon the sounds of the oral language. Letters and combinations of letters represent different sounds, or phonemes, and sequences of letters represent words. Although many children learn to spell pretty easily, it is actually a very abstract concept that presents great difficulty to some.

When will my child begin to write?

He will try some "pretend writing" very early, and progress from there. There are two phases of writing development that begin at about a year old and continue into kindergarten: Pre-Representation and Intentional Representation. "Writing" begins, of course, with scribbles, but then evolves into actual letters as the child becomes more aware of words and spelling. We don't expect preschoolers or kindergarteners to be able to spell many words except their names, but youngsters are very proud of their attempts at "writing."

During the **Pre-Representational** stage, infants and toddlers make marks with writing tools while trying to figure out how to hold and manipulate crayons, pencils and markers. Their marks are not intended for meaning; they are scribbles for the sake of scribbling. It is important, though, for the child to scribble like this in order to become dexterous enough to control a writing/drawing instrument when she wants to convey objects, people, letters and numbers. She will be astonished at the difference between markers and chalk, or crayons and paints. Children at this stage do not label their drawings; they just make marks because it's fun.

Before 3 years of age children actually understand the difference between drawing and writing. When they scribble a drawing they will tell you about it; when they scribble letters they will tell you what it says, even if it looks a lot like the scribbled drawing. Children begin by scribbling, often in a circular motion, then progress to horizontal scribbling, then individual units, letters, and the child's own name.

Children recognize their own name in writing before they can write it themselves, and many children first learn letter/sound relationships by knowing the sounds in their own name. Research has shown, in fact, that children who can write their names easily have better understanding of initial and final consonants and of the concept of "word."

Preschoolers who are at the beginning of the **Intentional Representation** stage make marks, often repeating the same marks, to convey meaning. They also enjoy telling people what they have drawn, sometimes using "words" in their drawings – not real words, but scribbles that look similar to letters. There is not really much detail in their drawings, though, or in their telling about the drawings.

Older preschoolers (around 4 years of age) are generally emerging into the later stage of **Intentional Representation**, which contains more actual symbols and more detail. Children who make these drawings usually tell what is happening in the picture, as well as who and where the people are. They also use marks that are more letter-like, and will "read" them to you. Some practiced words may even be spelled correctly, like "MOM," or "I LOVE YOU."

What skills will prepare my child to learn to spell?

Of course, acquiring good fine motor skills is necessary for the ability to hold and manipulate a pencil, crayon or marker. Having fun scribbling, drawing, painting, and any other activity that provides practice in manipulating a writing/drawing tool should be encouraged. Paper with and without lines should be available so your toddler can practice writing and drawing within a confined space, attempting to form letters from left to right on lines.

Studies have shown, however, that the best predictors of success in learning to spell are phonological awareness and print knowledge (See Chapter 8: Reading). This means that in order for parents and caregivers to support spelling development, they need to talk about words as they read to their babies and toddlers, and to demonstrate what reading is all about.

Can I teach my preschooler the sound/letter relationships of spelling?

You can, and should, point out the sounds and letters in words as you read to your child – not only books, but also cereal boxes, juice containers, street signs – anything available to read to your child. Don't expect her to catch on right away, though. It usually takes years of experience with listening, speaking and seeing written words for children to develop into spellers.

Knowing that words have a beginning and an ending is important for the understanding of spelling, but it is really a very abstract concept. Think about it. Say the word "yes" to yourself. It takes about a second to pronounce the word. Do you think a young child can discriminate a beginning (y), middle (e) and end (s) of that word in one second? Of course not. That requires quite a bit of phonemic awareness, which is a metalinguistic listening skill, in addition to the understanding that the squiggles on a page are actually symbols for each of the sounds.

Asking a toddler what sound is at the beginning of "bat" makes no sense at all to him. Is there a beginning, middle and end in a word that takes one second to pronounce? Your child will probably have no idea what you're talking about. When your child is around four, though, if you've focused on the metalinguistic activities listed in the previous chapter on reading, your child will be prepared to catch on to spelling and phonics as soon as he is ready. Begin to teach your child how to write some words that are important to him, and watch his efforts, enthusiasm and progress.

What will my child's beginning spelling look like?

There is actually a sequence for the development of spelling that has been documented in many studies. These are stages most often noticed in preschoolers:

1. The length of a word correlates with the size of the object. For example, the child thinks "mosquito" must be a short word because a mosquito is very small and that "cow" must be a very long word because cows are big.

2. The child is beginning to understand letter/sound correspondence and often uses single letters to represent a word, like "U" for "you" and "R" for "are."

3. Any sequence of letters is a word. Sometimes a child will see the first letter of her name in a word and think it's her name, or if she sees WTGOB she will assume it is a word.

4. When children begin to learn the sounds for some letters, they will try to spell a syllable with that letter, or with consonants only. For example, "come" might first be spelled as "K," then as "KM."

5. A child will often omit many middle letters of words, focusing on the beginning sounds, then on ending sounds. For example, "snow" might be spelled as "so" or "camp" might be spelled as "kp."

6. Children usually begin to spell words the way they pronounce them. She will spell "bath" as "baf" if that is the way she pronounces it.

Why is it so difficult for my child to learn letter/sound correspondence?

Just think about how we try to introduce children to the sounds "made" by each letter of the alphabet. As was explained above, beginning and ending sounds are pretty abstract concepts, and a child has to be ready to associate specific "drawings" (letters) with them in order for this process to have meaning.

Phonemic and phonological awareness is a cognitive developmental process which prepares the child to learn the alphabet letters as symbols of sounds. Then he also has to discover that there is not an exact correspondence, but a range of sounds for each letter. Since a child's brain is constantly searching for patterns, it is also finding and using these auditory patterns to associate with visual symbols. Many of these patterns are discovered through phonemic and phonological awareness activities.

When your child begins to experiment with letter/sound correspondences for spelling, though, it is very likely that you will think she is more incorrect than she actually is. Because you already know how to spell words, you probably disregard many of the sounds and patterns that you hear. You might think you hear specific sounds in words because you know how they are spelled. (This was also explained in Chapter 2: Articulation and Phoneme Development) For example, there is no /t/ sound in "kitten" the way we usually pronounce that word. You probably think there is a /t/ in the middle of the word, but it is actually a plosive sound made in the back of the throat. Say "kitten" in a sentence and listen to the way you pronounce it.

More difficulty is noticed when we begin to teach children the sounds corresponding to letters. We usually tell them the letter, and then the sound in isolation. In fact, though, it is very difficult to pronounce phonemes by themselves, when they are not in a word. For example, when we try to pronounce the /b/ phoneme in isolation, it often sounds more like "buh" (two sounds – /b/ + "uh"). That is because we have to produce some sound from our vocal cords in order to voice the /b/ sound. Otherwise we would be producing a /p/, the unvoiced sound. However, there is no "buh" in "bat," and children know that (otherwise it would be pronounced "buh-at"). So it is important to concentrate on pronouncing the sound as purely as possible (it takes some practice to be able to do this). We frequently confuse children because of our own perception of phonics and sound symbol relationships.

What will preschool teachers do to prepare my child for spelling?

Preschool teachers will most likely teach the alphabet, have a "word of the day" beginning with the letter they are teaching, point out words by "sounding them out," and use other such strategies to teach sound/letter correspondence. Teachers of young children encourage them to spell words the way they sound in order for the child to be able to pair writing with speaking: if she can say it, she can write it. This type of early spelling is often referred to as "invented spelling," but it might also be called transitional or temporary spelling. Children should know that this is beginning spelling, that it is a good start (real spelling is not reinvented by each person), and that they will get better at it as they are taught the adult way.

It is important for parents and teachers to understand how phonemes are produced and how the child's perception of sound sequences is developed in order to make sense of children's early attempts at spelling. It is easier to instruct a child to get from transitional spelling to the correct spelling of a word if he is shown how the word sounds, and then is lead to a better spelling. For example, if a child spells "big" as "pig," it may be that he is whispering the word to himself, so he *isn't* voicing the /b/. To him it sounds like a /p/. Watch your child try to spell words and listen to what he is doing. Preschool teachers should also be doing this. This will give you and his teacher the clues you need to help him to become a writer.

After my child can spell some words, will she be able to write sentences?

That depends on you. Since most preschoolers and kindergarteners don't really know what a sentence is, they need to be taught through modeling. You can show your child how to write short (two to three words) sentences word by word and then help her to write a sentence that she has spoken. She probably won't know what a sentence is yet, but if you keep using the word "sentence," she will eventually catch on.

Also be a role model as a writer. Even when you are just making notes for yourself (often in short sentence form), point out what you are writing and why, and be enthusiastic about its purpose: "Now I'll remember to get everything we need at the store," or "Mommy is going to send a nice email to Aunt Judy to thank her for bringing us that delicious cake!" Read some of your notes, emails, etc. to her so she will realize how easy it is.

Even if your child is able to write short sentences with you at home or in preschool, she still might have difficulty doing so in first or second grade. Some children can speak much better than they can write because the writing process involves the performance of many skills at once: generating ideas, formulating grammatical sentences, organizing and sequencing, sounding out, spelling, concentrating, planning grasping and pencil movements, and remembering the thoughts to be communicated. On the other hand, some children can write better than they can speak because of factors like the ability to edit and revise, to think slowly, and to organize before expressing thoughts in sentences. So whether your child finds speaking or writing easier, your job of helping her write sentences is to give her a great start – especially by showing her how writing can help her in so many ways.

If a family does not speak the "standard" dialect of English, will that affect a child's learning to spell?

As was mentioned previously, babies are born with the ability to hear differences in sounds, so they learn the accent or dialect of their environment as they learn to speak. By the time they are beginning to spell, however, they also must think about the sounds in words – a metalinguistic activity. In some families a "pin" (pen) is for writing, or a "caught" (cot) is a portable bed, or the sun sets in the "wes" (west). Parents, teachers and caregivers who are aware of these differences between pronunciation and spelling can make it fun for children to start discovering this on their own, another important metalinguistic development. When you are reading, making grocery lists, or labeling household items, point out the differences between your pronunciation and the spelling of the word. It will make your child aware of differences in spelling and pronunciation – and we have plenty of them in English!

SHARING THE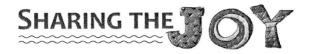

- ♥ Have your child match plastic alphabet letters by finding all the As and putting them in a container, then all the Bs, and so forth.

- ♥ Put alphabet puzzles together as a good way to notice how letters are formed.

- ♥ Provide a toddler-size easel or large pad of paper that can stand up, non-toxic paints, and paint brushes with short handles for your child. Also set up an art table with newspapers or an old shower curtain to cover it.

- ♥ Notice how your toddler draws and paints, and provide some guidance with holding brushes, crayons, markers, etc. Ask her to tell you about it.

- ♥ Write your toddler's name, and other words, lightly on lined paper. Have her trace her name, then copy it when she is ready.

- ♥ Demonstrate how to form letters and have your child imitate your motions. Describe what you are doing: "A 'B' starts up here, then comes down. Then we make a loop from the top, into the center, and another loop to the bottom." This is better than just using dot-to-dot letters because it also teaches direction.

- ♥ Display your child's artwork and writing. Show him that it is appreciated.

- ♥ Play "I'm thinking of a letter." Begin to write a letter of the alphabet, then have your child guess the letter –

continue with parts of the letter until he guesses it or until the whole letter is written.

♥ Create signs for creative play with your child: "Doctor," "Exit," "Sit Here," "Bakery," "Open" and "Closed" signs for stores.

♥ Make paper props with your child for imaginative play: airline tickets, play money, doctor's prescriptions, restaurant place mats.

♥ Use inch cubes (or something similar, like Legos) to represent each syllable of a few words of different lengths (like "pan," "oven" and "elephant"). Then say one of the words and ask your preschooler to point to which group of blocks that would be. Clap out syllables with her to see if she's right.

♥ Put out 4 Legos, 3 of one color and 1 of another color. Put 2 of the same together, and put the other 2 together. Say a pair of words beginning alike, like "**d**uck" and "**d**og." Ask your child to choose the pair of Legos that goes with that. Continue by saying more word pairs, some beginning alike and some beginning with different sounds, like "turtle" and "fox." This is a great activity for phonemic awareness.

♥ Have your child help you with grocery lists as you write the items for her to see. "Sound out" each word as you print it.

♥ Have your child help you with grocery lists as you write the items for her to see.

♥ Play "First Sound – First Letter": Ask your 4-year-old to tell you the first sound in a word (like *big*), then the

first letter (B). This helps to teach the difference between sounds and letters for reading and writing.

♥ Make a category book with magazine pictures: pictures
of animals, pictures of vehicles, pictures of furniture,
etc. Write the names of the items next to them. Ask
your child to find the names of the items that begin
with a certain letter and "read" them to you.

♥ Make a category book (as above) with your 4-year-old,
but only put a picture of the name of the category (like
a lion for animals). Have your child name as many
items in the category as he can, and print them under
the picture. Then name an item and have him find the
word by looking at the beginning letter.

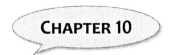

CHAPTER 10

Numbers and Math: Learning Numerical Concepts

Parents and preschool teachers often think of beginning mathematics as only counting and recognizing numbers. Mathematics, however, encompasses so many concepts: shapes (geometry), patterns (algebra), number operations (adding, subtracting, multiplying and dividing), spatial navigation (take two steps backwards), mapping (making visual representations of their classroom or bedroom) and even data analysis (watching progress, keeping charts).

Remember also that mathematics is language. It has its own vocabulary, semantic concepts, grammar, and relationships. We have to make inferences in math, associate and classify knowledge, and use the vocabulary and grammar of both math and non-math language in order to be successful in learning, talking about, and using mathematics. You already know that parents and caregivers need to stimulate all aspects of language, so be sure not to forget to stimulate in your child the language of numerosity, quantity, measurement, spatial awareness and logical thinking.

Are babies learning math?

Of course. And – this may surprise you – one of the first ways babies are introduced to math is through music. It has been shown that introducing young children to various types of music may have a very positive effect on the learning of mathematical concepts. Music inherently illustrates rhythm, tempo, changes in volume, harmony, sequencing, counting and patterning. Parents usually engage with babies in musical patterns in the form of rocking and patting, and in singing songs like "Twinkle Twinkle Little Star" while bouncing baby on their knee or rocking to the beat. Later, children's games like Patty-Cake teach children to keep a beat, patting hands together on the first beat of a sequence.

Besides developing skills through music, infants can also discriminate quantities – which plays an important role in the understanding of numbers. There are indications that very young infants can discriminate one dot from more than one dot on a paper. This is called *subitizing*, the ability to perceive a quantity, like three, and to differentiate it from another quantity without actually counting. So your baby's brain is figuring out numbers and quantity right from the beginning.

What kinds of toys will help my baby learn math?

Plastic shape puzzles are great for toddlers. Many studies have focused on shape composition as being significant in the development of math skills. Young children first manipulate shapes independently, but they do not flip or manipulate them to fit into a puzzle hole. They also do not put shapes together to form different shapes or pictures. After a while they are able to manipulate shapes to fit into a puzzle, but on a trial-and-error basis. Of course, children eventually learn to manipulate shapes purposefully, and even to make pictures with the shapes.

Colorful blocks are also wonderful for teaching spatial awareness. Playing with blocks is not only fun, but it develops important concepts needed to succeed at mathematical thinking: patterning, estimation, measurement, visualization, symmetry, part-whole relationships and balance. Think about how building with blocks involves spatial imagination – What am I going to build? How far away from each other should these blocks be to build a bridge? Do I have another block that looks like this for the other side? Since studies have shown that visual-spatial deficit is a major indicator of mathematical disability, it is an important skill to encourage while you and your child have fun playing with blocks.

An easy way to develop this skill with blocks is to train your child to imitate block designs, which requires focus on particulars of the design or pattern. First, give yourself and your child similar groups of blocks. Put a red block on the table and instruct your child to do the same. Then put a blue block next to it. Show your child how to do the same so that hers is a mirror image of yours. Then add another block to the design and have your child copy that. When your child does this easily, add two blocks at a time. This game can be repeated frequently, always adding more blocks at a time and making more complex structures. It is an active and strategic way to teach your child to envision parts and wholes simultaneously, a very important concept for mathematics.

When I teach my toddler to count, will she know what the numbers mean?

Once your toddler has memorized the number sequence to about "five," she will be ready to understand that the numbers actually symbolize quantity. "One" is the first she will understand, then "two." Once she understands the concept of "three" she is ready to begin counting with the one-to-one relationship of number to object. There is a strong correlation between number knowledge and vocabulary knowledge; children who have a larger vocabulary understand that words, including number words, have meaning. In fact, both semantic and morphological skills are important. Number concepts can be accelerated by the knowledge of the plural "s" marker in English (three apples) – one vs. many.

Another way to make numbers meaningful is to use numbers when reading stories to your child. If he can recognize objects that are named in stories and conversations, numbers will add even more meaning. While reading a story, you might say, "Look at the mommy duck and her three babies" or "Oh! Now there are four elephants!" and baby can focus on the elephants as well as the number of elephants standing in the water.

Parents, caregivers and preschool teachers who use a variety of new vocabulary with children should interject number words frequently. It has even been suggested that early learning of mathematical concepts is as great a predictor of academic success as early literacy skills. Many school-age children who demonstrate language difficulties also demonstrate more difficulties with numerical problems. So encouraging vocabulary and number sense together is an easy and effective way to give your child a head start.

What are the first mathematical skills my child will develop?

He will begin with the concept of *numerosity* – the understanding of quantity and measurement, which begins within the first year. Although 6-month-old infants cannot discriminate numerical differences between sets of dots (e.g., 8 vs. 12 dots), remarkably, 10-month-old infants are able to do so.

The concept of numerosity includes the understanding and use of many forms of numbers and their relationships to each other:

- ➢ Counting
- ➢ One-to-one correspondence
- ➢ Number words (one, six, three million)
- ➢ Numerals (4, 10, 300)
- ➢ Patterns on dice, cards and dominoes

➢ Detecting patterns (1 big, 1 little, 2 big, 2 little, 3 big …)
➢ Arithmetical procedures (addition, multiplication, subtraction, division)
➢ Geometric reasoning (identifying shapes, matching them, and fitting them together)
➢ Sets and subsets
➢ Fractions (¾, ⅔)
➢ Greater than and less than
➢ Logic (If A, then B)
➢ Reading and writing numbers
➢ Roman numerals (IV, X, XXVII)
➢ Sequencing

And more …

Children begin their acquaintance with numbers by hearing caregivers count with them – "one," "two," "three," "four," … after the child has already been introduced to the concept of numerosity. This, of course, is rote learning by memorizing the string of number words. But soon a child will associate the number words with actual quantities. During this important stage, memorization of numbers can be learned more easily if the speaker also uses some prosody, or a sing-songy way of saying the words. It makes it enjoyable, like a game or a song.

At about two years of age your child will begin to memorize the basic sequence of number words ("one," "two," "three"), and in preschool she should be able to count all the way to 20, a prediction of math success in the first grade.

When will my child be able to count objects?

Three-year-olds can generally understand the difference between "one" and "two," and many know that "seven" or "eight" mean more, but are generally able to count only two objects with one-to-one correspondence. By the end of the third year, however, most children will be able to count out a small number of items.

Many four-year-olds can solve counting problems like coloring in a certain number of squares on a grid to make different shapes with that number of squares. They can do this as an individual effort and in a group, helping each other to figure out additional shapes that can be made. However, although your child may be able to count small groups of objects or squares, he may be inconsistent in doing so. By five he will actually begin to add small numbers by counting all items, but he still might not always know that numerals label exact quantities. It often depends upon the task.

When will my child begin to add numbers of items?

Researchers have found that if an item is added to a group, a toddler is very likely to prefer any new label, whether it is the correct one or not. But between three and four years she will understand that if one object is added to a small set of objects the number of the set changes. With large quantities, though, "a lot" still remains "a lot." Most four-year-olds will count on their fingers, and will count to about twenty. By five they will also understand that the number word for a set of objects will change if one is added or removed, even with groups of objects larger than they can count.

The development of adding numbers usually begins with the child counting a set of objects, then counting the next set of objects, and finally counting all of them from the first to the last (1,2,3 – 1,2,3,4 – 1,2,3,4,5,6,7). Eventually the child will come to realize that she can continue counting from the end of the first set (the number 3) and just continue to the end of the second set (4,5,6,7).

When young children are asked "how many" (e.g., "How many dogs are in the park?"), if they know how to count, they will begin counting. The child might not know, however, that the last number they say is the correct answer for "how many," especially if he does not have a good grasp of the concept of "two" and "three." Once a child understands the concept of "four," though, he is on his way to understanding that adding an object means a group of objects will be named by a larger number. By five he may even be able to go forward in counting on a number line, or understand that taking one object away means going backwards on the number line, although he probably won't yet know which number is "six cows take away one cow."

After he begins to understand quantity, will my child know "more" and "less"?

"More" is often an early word, and many children use it to ask for second helpings and additional amounts ("more juice," "more tickle"). Children as young as three often compare amounts, and even talk about the comparisons with each other. At snack time Charlie might say, "I have this much more cereal than you," illustrating with his hands. Amy might ask Kevin for the small blocks he is playing with. When Kevin gives her only three, she might complain, "I want all of them!" showing her knowledge of the part-whole relationship. They probably won't use the word "less," though, until 4 or 5 years of age.

How does recognizing patterns relate to math?

We often don't think of math as involving patterns, but the pattern of adding one number at a time illustrates counting; the pattern of skipping numbers demonstrates odd and even numbers; the pattern of multiplying a number by itself results in squaring and cubing. Patterns can be found everywhere, especially in nature: the songs of birds, symmetry of leaves, butterfly wings, and footprints on the beach of a dog walking next to his owner. Once your child learns to look for patterns, she will also begin to see relationships between numbers – and that's what math is really all about.

How can I show my child different uses of numbers every day?

Let's think about some of the ways in which numbers are embedded in our everyday lives:

➢ Page numbers in books and magazines
➢ TV channels
➢ Money
➢ Time
➢ Dates
➢ Recipes
➢ Body weight
➢ Sharing equally

And more …

And not only do we count objects, but we can also count things that are audible (beats in a measure), tactile (number of rough edges) and thoughts (three wishes).

Parent and caregiver interaction with children about numeric and spatial concepts has an unquestionable effect on children's development of math skills. Children should be given many opportunities to think about numbers and to make estimations so they become much more intuitive about numbers. Talk to your child about what he is doing while playing with blocks or other spatial manipulatives. Encourage him to talk to himself while solving spatial problems. (stacking blocks, building bridges, etc.) Your "thinking aloud" will help him learn to think about what he is doing. ("Hmmm. I wonder how many more blocks we'll need to reach the table," or

"How many of these cups can we fill with this sand?") You can also model by stating the intent of the activity ("We're going to make a path we can walk on.") and the next step needed for the task. ("We need to see how many of this size we have left.") Estimates of the numbers of blocks needed can even be written on cards so the child will know how close he came with his guess.

What kind of math will my child be learning in preschool?

She should be hearing and learning the language of mathematics throughout the day. The amount of daily "math talk" used by preschool teachers greatly affects a child's knowledge of numerosity:

"Let's count how many children are here today." (counting people)

"I'm going to clap three times, then you can go to your seat." (counting auditory information)

"Let's see how many apples we have." (counting objects)

"Bobby and Jesse can share these equally" (division; equivalence)

"Three people say yes, five people say no. Which group has more people?" (non-equivalence)

"If you have a seven, put a chip on it." (number symbols)

"We have to wait till March 17th. Look at the calendar. Today is March 12th." (nominative sequencing)

"I'll read half the book today and half tomorrow." (fractions)

"If we take three beans from these six, how many do we have left?" (calculation)

The act of verbalizing problems, at home and in preschool, is adding to the child's repertoire of semantic concepts that will help her communicate and learn. Preschool teachers should listen as each child verbalizes – it helps adults to judge how she is solving problems. Besides teaching some basic counting, adding, and subtracting, preschool teachers should teach much more than formulas. Math is thinking. Can you imagine anyone comprehending what they've read if they have only been trained in grammar and spelling? It's the same with math, which is definitely not only numbers and calculations. Comprehension is key, and parents and preschool teachers have the opportunity to model and encourage numerical problem solving and comprehension throughout the day.

What other skills will help my child learn mathematics?

There is a seemingly non-math skill that many studies have found affects both social skills and mathematical development. It is called *executive functioning*. Executive functioning, or *executive control*, is actually a number of cognitive abilities:

➢ the ability to focus on goal-directed behaviors
➢ the ability to inhibit/control compulsive behavior
➢ the ability to attend well
➢ the ability to remember what needs to be done to accomplish a task (also called *working memory*)

Since mathematical tasks are complex, they require us to hold many bits of information in memory while determining strategies and monitoring progress. This requires, as you might expect, quite a bit of focus, attention and patience. Watch your child as she attempts to solve problems. Does

182

she become easily frustrated, or can she stick with a task to completion?

As was mentioned above, children who demonstrate good spatial skills also seem to have a better sense of mathematics. This is often demonstrated when a child examines details of objects, which allows her to use informal measurements to solve spatial problems. She might figure out how many Legos she will need to build a certain structure, or she might decide if she will have enough time to draw a picture before leaving for Grandma's house. See if your child automatically categorizes shapes, putting all the circles into one pile. Notice whether she puts five inch cubes on a paper with the numeral 5 all by herself. Watch her set the table with just the right number of dishes and spoons for her four dolls. Watch as your two children stand next to each other to see who is taller. These are all clues you can use to determine whether your child is on the right track for learning mathematical concepts.

SHARING THE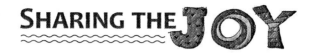

- ♥ Count toys while putting them away.

- ♥ Sort toys: cars, dolls, animals, etc. Make cards with numbers and have your child label each set.

- ♥ Ask which is larger? Largest? Smaller? Smallest?

- ♥ Look for things with shapes: circles, squares, triangles.

- ♥ Make a "puzzle" on a piece of paper by tracing around shapes of small household items. Then put the items in front of your child so she can put each onto its shape on the paper.

- ♥ Ask, "How many corners on this shape? How many edges?"

- ♥ Match straws to juice cartons for one-to-one correspondence.

- ♥ Sort silverware into sets: forks, knives, spoons.

- ♥ Fold napkins into rectangles and triangles.

- ♥ Line up pots by size: largest to smallest.

- ♥ Find out how many cups it takes to fill a pot.

- ♥ Sort laundry: socks, shirts, pants, towels.

- ♥ Count stairs as you go up.

- ♥ Name places seen from the car in the order in which they were seen. (First we saw _____, then we saw _____.)

- ♥ Find things that come in twos (pairs): feet, eyes, ears, shoes, socks.

- ♥ Find things that come in fives: fingers, toes, gloves.

- ♥ Give choices: "You may have two cookies. Would you like the round ones or the square ones?"

- ♥ Put small objects on number cards: 3 rubber bands, two paper clips, 5 pencils, etc.

- ♥ Take objects out of "Mystery Bag" for classification by function. (different kinds of flatware, drawing tools, hair accessories …)

- ♥ Take one bite of food after each number: "One!" "Two!" "Three!" "Four!"

- ♥ "Let's put 5 chocolate chips in each cookie."

- ♥ Play "How Many Did I Take?" with various objects.

- ♥ Teach comparatives. ("Let's get a *large* bowl of popcorn, not a *small* bowl.")

- ♥ Add descriptive words (long, short, fat, thin, large, small) and comparatives (longest, shortest, fattest, thinnest, largest, smallest) when asking your child to find objects for a shapes game.

- ♥ Use geoboards to make different shapes and to name them. Also make the shapes oriented in different directions – flipped sideways, pointing the opposite way, etc.

- ♥ Deconstruct cereal boxes to see how many rectangles make up the box. Then tape them back together into its original 3-dimensional container.

- ♥ Play "Simon Says" with positional words like above, below, beside, between, under, next to, inside, outside, etc. with shapes: "Simon says put the triangle between the little circle and the big circle."

♥ Use positional words when talking about daily tasks. ("Put the napkin beside the fork," "Tuck the sheet under the mattress," "Put the top on the jar.")

♥ Count how many steps it takes to get from one place to another, like from the sofa to the refrigerator. Take guesses, then see if you're close.

♥ Count people in the family, then figure out how many hands and how many feet are in the family.

♥ Talk aloud when helping your child share equally. "Let's see how many grapes Charles will get and how many John will get." Together count the grapes on the bunch, then divide them equally: "One, one, two, two, …"

♥ Play "Finish the Pattern" with colored inch cubes (red, red, blue, red, red, blue, red, red, …) or any other small items (fork, spoon, fork, spoon, fork, spoon, …) Also continue patterns with words (bear, cat, sheep, bear, cat, sheep, bear …), musical tones (sing the same 3-note sequence twice, then have your child continue), claps, etc.

♥ Play "Do What I Do" with imitating patterns: sway, hop, tap on a pot or the table to a beat. Change the beat. Go faster, then slower.

♥ Count the number of syllables in words by clapping them out. This also teaches metalinguistics (what a word is and what a syllable is).

♥ Line up items on a table to see which is longer and longest (fork, spoon, spatula, rolling pin, etc.), shorter and shortest. Then introduce another object and have your child put it in the right place according to length.

♥ Paste small magazine pictures of objects in categories onto pages (trees, building, flowers, food, etc.). Arrange the pages from the smallest number of items to the largest. Write each number at the top of each page. Then cut out another group of pictures in one category. Count the items and have your child figure out where it goes in the sequence of pages.

♥ Play "speed Dominoes" by putting all the 2s together, all the 3s together, etc. without counting the dots (a good way to teach subitizing).

♥ Play a concentration game with Dominoes to match ones that are the same. Sometimes have the Dominoes placed on the table/floor vertically, sometimes horizontally.

♥ Make Bingo cards with different arrangements of dots in each square. Say a number and have your child put a candy on the square. Later hold up a card with the number written on it rather than saying the number out loud.

♥ Play "Let's see how far we can count." Begin counting in unison with your child. When you get to numbers she doesn't know, emphasize the first number of each 10 ("**thirty**!"), then emphasize the numbers 1 to 9 to help him understand the pattern: "thirty-**one**, thirty-**two**, thirty-**three** ..."

♥ Put out some cards all with the same number on them and one with a different number. Ask your child which one does not belong with the others.

♥ Ask your child to find different shapes in the environment, both inside and outside. ("Look! The fridge is shaped like a rectangle." "The wheels on the car look like big circles!")

♥ Take photos of objects that are different shapes and organize them into *circle, square, rectangle, triangle,* etc. folders (can also be computer folders).

♥ Make comparisons with shapes: "The donut circle is a lot *smaller than* the ball circle. Can we find a circle that is even *smaller*? Yes! This button!"

♥ Use pipe cleaners, toothpicks, straws and Play-Doh to make shapes and then ask how each can be turned into another shape. Also notice how shapes can be combined, like two triangles making a square or rectangle.

♥ Name 3-dimensional shapes for your child: sphere, cube, cylinder, cone.

♥ Estimate, then count: people in a room, books on the table, spoons in the drawer.

♥ Teach *more* and *fewer*. (Are there fewer horses or fewer riders? More?)

♥ Compare pots and containers: Which holds more? Which holds less?

♥ Count sets and subsets: "Let's count the M&Ms. One, two, three, four, five, six, seven. How many are blue? How many are red? If we add the blue ones to the red ones, how many do we have?"

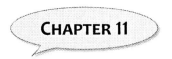

Learning with TV and Other Electronic Media

Should my toddler watch TV?

There have been many recent studies about the effect of television viewing on young children. Results of these studies vary somewhat. But most are in agreement for one conclusion: the most important activity encouraging language development is child/parent interaction. Research has focused on the effects of television and video on cognitive development, attention, language, executive function, and obesity. Many children who begin watching TV and playing video games early are those children who, when they are older, demonstrate what the medical field is now calling "Electronic Screen Syndrome," characterized by mental (disruptive behavior, agitation, lack of focus) and physical (sleep deprivation, lethargy, obesity) impairments. These will be discussed below.

Should my child be learning from educational TV?

Before the age of 2 children's brains do not learn from objects moving on a screen, and their receptive language skills (listening and understanding) are not developed sufficiently to comprehend the programs. Some studies have called this a "video deficit" of toddlers. Preschoolers and young children above the age of 3, though, can be entertained at times by programs that move slowly enough to give their brains time to process information. Many educational TV programs include actors, often dressed as characters, interacting with each other, so TV programs that mimic this social interaction are sometimes successful at teaching concepts to preschoolers. Toddlers, on the other hand, have learned that their primary source of information is other people; they use social cues such as eye gaze, gestures, and the recognition of new words to learn new information as they themselves interact with others. Since the movement of people on TV do not evoke a response from toddlers, they rarely regard them as viable sources of information.

Programs like Sesame Street, Dora the Explorer, or Bill Nye the Science Guy include repetition of ideas and time for information processing. But if an adult sits with the child, asks the child questions, points out interesting facts, and even pauses the show to explain, discuss, or paraphrase, the child will learn much more from the program. The key is adult/child interaction. Ask your child questions like, "How do you think he did that?" or "How do you think scientists figured that out?" Many educational programs also offer online questions that parents can ask their children to spark conversation during and after TV viewing. Engage your child in learning, and eventually your child will be able to critique TV shows and know which are mere nonsense, or just boring, and which are interesting and worthwhile.

Can TV or other media help my child's language development and literacy?

Video might be a source of entertainment for toddlers, but there is little evidence that it teaches language – and it certainly doesn't teach babies to read. In fact, most children under two years cannot comprehend the message of videos at all. Even children who were presented with a normal version and a distorted version of Teletubbies, a program for young children, could not distinguish between the two versions. The most significant predictor of language and vocabulary development is the amount of time a child is read to and her positive interactions with caregivers, not a DVD program that convinces parents it is what they must use for their baby's language.

It is rather strange, in fact, that some videos are geared toward very young infants, although these infants have very poor visual acuity, depth perception and color vision. Also, the 2-D format does not fit their developmental level as do 3-dimensional interactions with caregivers. Some research, in fact, has suggested that early exposure to videos actually results in lower overall language scores on cognitive tests.

It is also interesting that DVDs marketed toward infants and toddlers proclaiming increased vocabulary, cognitive or reading skills, rarely use social interaction between child and caregiver. This seems strange given the necessity for children to experience developmentally appropriate interactions. Some infant videos even contain onscreen print, a strange strategy for teaching given the fact that infants cannot read. So can parents use TV or video to develop language skills? Not much. Interacting with your child, asking questions and explaining words and content, what we call "instructional scaffolding," is the way to develop your child's language and to continue to build a healthy child-parent relationship.

There have been many programs marketed to parents claiming to make their child a genius or an early reader who will excel in school and continue to learn quickly. Parents must beware, however, of programs or systems that are not based upon how children learn. These very often are not only useless for teaching babies and toddlers, they can actually be harmful if they are replacing learning from parents and caregivers. If you are knowledgeable about child development, you are unlikely to be fooled into buying programs to speed up your child's learning process.

Remember that infancy and early childhood is a critical time for brain development. Just as one needs to practice throwing a ball in order to learn that skill, a baby needs to practice thinking, problem solving, changing opinions and communicating thoughts and needs in order to become a skilled thinker. Unstructured play, with or without an adult, will allow the child to explore, discover, and learn. Interacting with others will teach the child to communicate, to think and solve problems, and to learn language. Don't rely on any video programs to teach your child anything as well as you can.

Could watching TV or videos hurt my child in any way?

Some studies have discovered that infants who watched DVDs had poorer language development (especially 12-month-old infants who watched TV for two hours a day). When infants engage in positive interactions with parents and caregivers at times when they are not viewing the videos, however, they are probably less likely to be adversely affected by the media. The key seems to be in the amount of time viewing vs. the time interacting with adults. Very little, or no, viewing time seems to be best.

It has also been shown that preschool children who watch television programs that are directed toward adults can exhibit lower cognitive functioning and executive functioning (memory, attention, self-control and emotions) at age 4. Since more TV and video watching is associated with less mother-child interaction in such activities as book reading, and even playing with toys, it sometimes has a disruptive effect on parent-child relationships – especially on forming secure, loving relationships. Adult programs also make no sense to young children, and their content can often be cognitively confusing.

TV also frequently replaces physical activity and social contact with other children. Since so many children in the U.S. are overweight, physical activity and healthy eating are crucial.

Children who spend long hours in front of the TV eating unhealthy snacks (and watching commercials for "junk" food and beverages) are obviously at risk of becoming overweight, or even obese. Playing with others develops social skills and friendships that are difficult to cultivate while watching TV.

Some studies have also suggested that watching TV or DVDs in infancy can actually lead to ADHD because of over-stimulation of the developing brain. For example, researchers have found that just 9 minutes of watching fast-paced cartoons has affected the executive functioning of 4-year-olds. This has been refuted, however, by other research, which found only a correlation with ADHD for children who viewed TV for more than 7 hours per day. Furthermore, other researchers have suggested that some parents who use TV as a "babysitter" do so because their child is already more active and has an exhausting (to the parent) temperament. So this is at least something we need to think about.

It has also been illustrated that television viewing for infants and toddlers is sometimes associated with irregular sleep schedules, both at naptime and bedtime. Since a routinized sleep pattern is important for babies, parents should be aware of this when setting a schedule for baby's sleep.

Researchers have even studied the effect of TV background noise on young children. It has been estimated that the average child in the US is exposed to more than 230 minutes of background television per day. Preschoolers raised in an environment with constant TV background noise have scored lower on some psychological and cognitive tests. Other studies, however, have refuted this and have even suggested that background sounds may actually train some children to develop strategies for focusing in a noisier environment. This might be a result of individual differences, though, so it is best to see how your child reacts to the background sound of TV. If she seems disturbed at all, she may need a quieter environment in which to think, learn and relax.

Of course, whenever choosing TV programs or DVDs for your child it is important to be sure they are age appropriate. Exposure to adult-directed TV has been shown to lessen executive function and increase aggression, anxiety and hyperactivity in children. Remember that children do not need to be exposed to violence as a form of entertainment. Age appropriate TV programs can be entertaining, and even educational, when monitored carefully. Enjoy a little time in front of TV or videos with your child, but don't let them replace adult-child time, both active and quiet play time, and social activities.

Because of many recent studies of the effects of electronic media on children, The American Academy of Pediatrics guidelines suggest that televisions, computers and video should be avoided for children under the age of two. It also suggests that parents closely monitor all children's TV viewing and use of other media. Studies have been somewhat contradictory, but your knowledge about how language and learning develops will help you immensely in deciding how to handle your child's exposure to media.

SHARING THE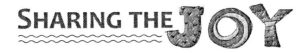

- ♥ Make sure that TV and/or other media is age-appropriate for your child.

- ♥ Interact with your little one during very limited TV or media for very young children. He probably won't learn much, but will enjoy the interaction.

- ♥ Limit TV for children 2 to 5 year – 1 hour or less per day is best.

- ♥ Watch TV or DVDs with your child and explain content and new words for vocabulary and interest.

- ♥ Ask your child questions about the content while viewing to keep her engaged and watching the program for answers to your questions.

- ♥ Talk about and review the program after watching, then again the next day.

- ♥ Take follow-up trips to the library to find books on the topic (even if they are picture books).

- ♥ Discuss TV advertising with your child and ask her if it made her want the product. Awareness should begin early.

- ♥ Be a role model for limiting TV time. Homes with fewer hours of TV watching tend to be more cognitively stimulating.

- ♥ Suggest playing outside, drawing, playing with toys and looking at books rather than watching TV. Share the joy with your healthy, energetic, creative child!

Appendix A

Disabilities Affecting
Speech and Language

If your child is diagnosed with any of the following disabilities, an Individual Educational Plan (IEP) might be developed by the special education team at your child's school. Use this only as a beginning guide. If you suspect that your child is not developing within normal limits in any way, please consult medical experts.

Most children, of course, develop speech and language just fine. But it is best for parents to be aware of symptoms of possible delays and disabilities – just in case. In this chapter you will find some basic information about a number of ways the development of speech and/or language can be compromised. If you are concerned because your child shows symptoms of something not being quite right, it is best to make an appointment for an evaluation by a speech-language pathologist. There is a range of normalcy, which has been emphasized in this book, but sometimes a child might show signs of delay that are outside of that range.

The descriptions in this chapter are very short summaries of various syndromes and impairments. The medical/educational team for your child (pediatrician, speech-language pathologist, audiologist, neurologist, etc.) will provide you with much more information, and it will be specific to your child.

Auditory Processing Disorder (APD)

Auditory processing disorder (APD), also referred to as central auditory processing disorder (CAPD), refers to difficulty for the brain to process auditory information. Some of the same characteristics are evident in children with APD as in children diagnosed with specific language impairment (SLI), so differential diagnosis is important.

Children with APD have no hearing loss, yet they have trouble understanding speech in noisy environments (auditory figure-ground difficulties), following directions, telling the difference between speech sounds, and learning to read and spell. Although a speech-language pathologist, a teacher, a pediatrician, or even a psychologist may suspect a child has APD, an actual diagnosis must be made by an audiologist. Usually a child must be at least 7 years of age for a diagnosis, but an audiologist can give suggestions for a younger child who is suspected of having APD. Treatment is highly individualized and is developed for a child's specific type of auditory disorder.

ADD/ADHD

Attention deficit hyperactivity disorder (ADHD) in young children is characterized by some of these behaviors:

- difficulty attending to tasks
- not listening or following directions
- fidgeting and squirming a lot
- running or climbing when asked to sit or listen
- interrupting
- pushing or pulling others
- bumping into other children frequently
- having difficulty sleeping

Sometimes ADHD affects a child's language development, especially social skills. Since children learn most social skills by observing those around him, lack of observation skills paired with impulsivity decreases a child's awareness of appropriate ways to communicate. Children with ADHD are also likely to exhibit learning and/or language disabilities. It is very difficult for a child's brain to attend to the words and structure of language when the brain is unable to focus and reflect. Attending to letter sounds and writing letters and numbers also require attention that may be difficult for the child. A speech-language pathologist will most likely work on a team (pediatrician, occupational therapist, and others) for a child with ADHD.

Autism Spectrum Disorder (ASD)

ASD is characterized by various degrees of difficulty with social interaction and verbal and non-verbal communication. It can also include repetitive behaviors that is described as self-stimulation, or "stimming," and inflexible adherence to routines. ASD can be classified as mild (previously referred to as Asperger's Syndrome) to more severe (autism or pervasive developmental disorder). Many people "on the spectrum" are very talented visually, academically or musically. It is also not uncommon for children with ASD to exhibit problems with coordination, and health issues (especially gastrointestinal disorders) are commonly present. Many more boys than girls are diagnosed with ASD (1 out of 42 boys and 1 out of 189 girls according to www.AutismSpeaks.org) and its numbers seem to be increasing each year.

The American Academy of Pediatrics recommends that children be screened for ASD at 18 and 24 months. If a parent or pediatrician suspects ASD, the child is generally then referred to an autism specialist for further assessment. If a child is found to have ASD, early intervention is crucial. This can include speech-language therapy, occupational therapy, medical and dietary treatments, and other interventions appropriate for the individual child.

Cerebral Palsy (CP)

Cerebral palsy (CP) is a neurological disorder that affects body movement and coordination. It is caused by brain injury before, during, or immediately after birth. A child with cerebral palsy will not be able to control his muscles, which will contract too much or too little, causing limbs to shake, tremble or writhe.

Cerebral palsy usually affects speech, so a child with CP should be assessed by a speech-language pathologist at or before the age of two, since that is the age when first words are spoken. Speech therapy will improve functioning of the lips, tongue, jaw and throat for articulation. Some children with CP also need language therapy, and some, those who have great difficulty with speech, may need to learn sign language or alternate forms of communication.

Childhood Apraxia of Speech (CAS)

Childhood apraxia of speech (CAS) is a neurological speech sound disorder in which an impairment of the movement of articulators (lips and tongue) causes difficulty producing sounds, syllables and words. Although a child with this disorder has difficulty with the exact movements of muscles needed for correct speech sounds and prosody, the difficulty in movement does not originate in the muscles; it originates in the part of the brain that controls the articulators. Sometimes the apraxia is genetic and heredity, and sometimes it can be caused by birth trauma, but it is more often idiopathic – of unknown cause.

Symptoms of CAS can include the following:

- decreased cooing or babbling as an infant
- late beginning speech with words that are missing sounds or are distorted

- trouble chewing and swallowing some foods
- understanding of language much better than speaking
- difficulty pronouncing longer words
- speech that is generally difficult to understand, especially for an unfamiliar listener
- speech sounds choppy and distorted
- articulation of sounds is inconsistent (i.e., not just a consistent lisp or w/r substitution)
- may or may not have difficulty with motor movement in other parts of the body

Apraxia usually results in delayed speech, and intelligibility is seriously compromised when the child speaks. You will know that your child's speech is delayed long before she enters kindergarten. A speech-language pathologist can determine whether your child has apraxia and can begin therapy even before your child is three years of age. Treatment should begin early so the child can begin to use his new way of speaking as soon as possible. The speech-language pathologist will most likely see the child 2 to 3 times per week at the beginning and will give instructions for home carryover.

Cleft Lip or Palate

It is estimated that 1 or 2 out of every 1000 babies will be born with a cleft lip or palate. The cleft is the result of the tissue of the lip or roof of the mouth failing to fuse together during the first 6 to 10 weeks of pregnancy. A cleft can be either unilateral or bilateral, and most children have surgery to repair the cleft within the first year or two. Parents won't have to look for symptoms of cleft lip or palate because it will be identified at birth.

Not all children with a cleft lip or palate will need speech therapy, but a speech-language therapist should monitor the child's development through early childhood.

Dysarthria

Dysarthria is a motor speech disorder affecting muscles of articulation: lips, tongue, vocal cords, and sometimes diaphragm. It is caused by damage to the brain, sometimes from birth trauma. Conditions such as cerebral palsy, muscular dystrophy, brain injury and multiple sclerosis are often accompanied by dysarthria.

Symptoms of dysarthria include the following:

- slurred or mumbled speech
- either slow or rapid speech
- limited tongue, lip or jaw movement
- abnormal pitch and/or rhythm
- speech that sounds either nasal or "stuffed up"

A speech-language pathologist can provide treatment goals for children exhibiting dysarthria to lessen its severity, even if the cause of the dysarthria will continue. Therapy will focus on what the child can do to make her speech more understandable to listeners.

Hearing Impairment

Some hospitals offer very sophisticated techniques for detecting congenital hearing loss. Baby's brain waves can show that baby is responding to auditory stimulation. If your hospital does not offer this type of testing it may be a year or more before you suspect that your baby might have a hearing loss. Also, many children have intermittent hearing loss: sometimes they hear fine, but at other times they don't. This is generally caused by ear infections. So being a good observer is important.

Parents need to be aware of signs of possible hearing impairment:

- babbles very little; may even "babble" with hands

- does not look at you while you speak
- does not respond to whispered speech
- does not change pitch and intensity when crying
- does not use any words by two years of age
- speaks loudly in a high-pitched voice
- does not attend to your voice or turn to look in your direction
- shows little interest in conversations
- distorts sounds in words when speaking

These might be indicators of hearing loss, but they also might indicate other types of language impairment mentioned in this section on disabilities.

Babies who are born with a hearing loss should be exposed to sign language as soon as possible. Language, as we know, is not only oral. Even hearing babies attend to our gestures and facial expressions as a very important part of the communicative process.

Intellectual Disabilities

An intellectual disability is characterized by limitations in intellectual functioning (generally an IQ score of 70 and below) and adaptive behavior (social and daily living skills). It affects learning, problem solving and reasoning, as well as speech and language. Down Syndrome is one cause of intellectual disability, but there are also many others. Many include specific physical characteristics that are present at birth, and diagnosis is early. Some children with an intellectual disability have significantly delayed language, so they may need to use sign language or augmentative communication devices. But many children will just need the services of a speech-language pathologist to improve the child's oral communication skills.

Language Delay or Specific Language Impairment (SLI)

There are many symptoms of language delay, but parents should be aware of any combination of these in order to consider a speech and language evaluation. Pediatricians can write a referral for your child, and your local school system can also schedule an evaluation. If your child needs therapy, an Individual Education Plan (IEP) can be developed even for very young children.

Symptoms of possible language delay:

- not babbling by the age of 15 months
- not speaking by age 2
- pointing to objects instead of asking with words by age 2
- difficulty in following simple directions
- not speaking in short sentences by age 3
- multiple articulation errors; difficult to understand

If you have been following the suggestions in the Sharing the JOY sections of this book and your child is not progressing as he should be, don't hesitate to get help. The sooner a problem is discovered the better his chance of overcoming any difficulties.

Language Learning Disabilities (LLD)

Children with language-based learning disabilities have difficulty with reading, spelling, and/or writing. If the disability mainly affects reading, it is sometimes labeled *dyslexia*. But learning disabilities, or language-based learning disabilities, often include difficulties with spoken language as well. Since young children are not expected to read or write well, it is often difficult to diagnose a learning disability in a preschooler. If a language-based learning disability is suspected, however, a speech-language pathologist can observe the child and formally assess some skills that might need remediation.

Early symptoms might include difficulties with the following:
* organizing thoughts (oral and/or written)
* decreased vocabulary ("stuff," or "that thing" rather than labels)
* finding the right word (word retrieval problems)
* understanding questions
* following directions
* remembering stories
* understanding stories
* remembering sequences of letters and/or numbers
* understanding directionality (writing letters left to right, holding a book right-side up)
* learning the alphabet
* learning letter sounds
* rhyming words
* spelling her name

Non-Verbal Learning Disorder (NVLD)

Non-verbal learning disorder is characterized by difficulty with social expression and interpretation (pragmatics) as well as reading comprehension and spatial awareness. It is usually diagnosed in elementary school, when children are expected to comprehend and interpret reading material. But there may be signs of NVLD in preschool, so parents who notice signs of it should focus on the development of pragmatic language skills.

Children with NVLD might exhibit the following behaviors:
* be awkward or clumsy (trouble with visual/spatial orientation)

- have difficulty retelling a story or relating events in an organized fashion
- have difficulty answering questions about a story that requires making inferences ("Why was mother so angry?")
- misunderstand facial expressions and body language of others
- seem not to be learning social appropriateness (in later years might lack social tact)
- may learn by rote, but have difficulty putting the learning into practice and applying rules
- have difficulty learning the physical layout of the preschool (how to get to the play yard, etc.)

If you have concerns about the possibility of your child having non-verbal learning disorder, you can mention this to his teacher when he begins kindergarten. If she notices a problem, she will probably recommend an observation by the school speech-language pathologist.

Selective Mutism

Children with selective mutism withhold speech in specific social situations, but do speak in others. It is not caused by a language delay or speech problem that makes oral communication difficult. Children with selective mutism may also exhibit shyness or social anxiety or withdrawal. A speech evaluation for selective mutism will consist of a hearing test, assessment of the physical speech mechanism, medical history, history of symptoms and of speech-language development, verbal and non-verbal language assessments, and questions about the family and environmental factors. A child with selective mutism will generally receive services from a speech-language pathologist and a psychologist, who will provide information and strategies to parents, caregivers and teachers.

Sensory Processing Disorder (SPD)

We use sensory-motor integration, or processing, in order to be able to perform more than one activity at once – like watching TV, sitting upright on the sofa and drinking lemonade – using all of our senses together without having to expend a lot of energy. This is something we rarely think about because daily actions like walking, listening to music, and watching where we're going just come naturally to most of us. It is estimated, however, that SPD may affect as many as 1 in 20 children.

These are some symptoms of sensory processing disorder in toddlers:

- irritable when dressing; uncomfortable wearing clothes
- difficulty playing with toys that require dexterity, like building blocks or coloring
- difficulty shifting from one activity to another
- extremely active or constantly moving
- speech is difficult to understand
- stumbles over words or has unusual rhythm of speech
- does not seem to understand directions
- spins around in circles frequently
- delayed in crawling, standing or walking
- resists being held and cuddled
- doesn't like the texture of many foods
- is easily startled
- overreacts to sensory stimulation: noise, smells, taste, touch, visually busy spaces
- seems clumsy or awkward
- hits other children when they touch him

If your child is diagnosed with sensory processing disorder, he will most likely need to see an occupational therapist, and possibly a speech-language pathologist. It is common for specialists to work as a team for remediation of such disabilities.

Stuttering

No doubt parents will read a number of conflicting articles about the causes and nature of stuttering, as well as some very diverse "treatments" and "cures" for stuttering. Having knowledge about the disorder along with some skepticism about the "latest cures," however, is necessary in order to get the appropriate help for a child who stutters.

When children are just developing speech and language, they exhibit normal disfluencies. Nothing as complex as speech and language could be learned without stumbling. Normal disfluencies might include repetition of sounds, words and phrases, and stopping and starting over. These normal behaviors, though, are not accompanied by struggle or frustration.

By the time a child is 4 years of age, and often younger, a child who stutters can already be exhibiting avoidance behaviors and can exhibit stress in speaking situations.

These behaviors can be indicative of actual stuttering:

- repeating syllables or sounds with struggle
- prolonging sounds or syllables
- trying to "get the sound out"
- exhibiting struggle behavior or tension
- changing volume or pitch
- showing frustration while speaking
- exhibiting facial grimacing
- hitting his body, tapping his feet, jiggling, etc.
- having a family history of stuttering

A speech-language pathologist can diagnose stuttering, provide therapy, and consult with family members about what to do while speaking with and listening to the child. There are also very good resources for parents at www.stutteringhelp.org.

Velopharyngeal Insufficiency (VPI)

Velopharyngeal insufficiency is a disorder resulting from the improper closing of the back of the soft palate during speech, resulting in nasal sounds and difficulty with plosive sounds like /p/, /b/, /t/ and /g/. Air can frequently be heard escaping from the nose, and sometimes squeaks or snorts are evident, during speech. VPI can be a result of cleft palate (including repaired), adenoidectomy, or unknown causes. A speech-language pathologist can diagnose VPI in conjunction with an otolaryngologist (ear, nose and throat doctor). VPI can be treated with surgery, an oral appliance, and speech therapy.

Voice Disorders

Voice disorders are medical conditions that affect pitch, volume and voice quality. Some parents think that a child with a hoarse or raspy voice just "sounds that way." But children often abuse their voices by talking loudly or yelling, or otherwise misusing their vocal cords, and that can cause a voice disorder like vocal nodules or polyps, or other types of dysphonia.

If your child exhibits these symptoms, an examination of his vocal cords by a laryngologist is needed before speech therapy can begin:

- ◆ hoarseness
- ◆ breathiness
- ◆ a "rough" or "scratchy" voice
- ◆ decreased pitch range
- ◆ frequent sore throats

If the laryngologist discovers a vocal cord disorder, medical treatment will precede speech therapy. Once speech therapy begins, the speech-language pathologist will prescribe ways for the child and family to continue on a path of vocal health.

APPENDIX B

Choosing a Preschool or Caregiver

Now that you understand the importance of language development, you realize that it is imperative to choose a preschool or caregiver who also understands all aspects of early language. Of course, whoever you choose must also be enthusiastic about caring for and working with your child, and must want to work closely with you to encourage your child to become an excellent communicator.

Most of the characteristics discussed below pertain to both preschool settings and to caregivers who may be working with your child only, or with a very small group of toddlers or preschoolers. If you hire a caregiver, or "babysitter," (or if a friend or relative cares for your child), some of these requirements, like certification and professional development will not apply. Please read and think about this section carefully, though, so you can become a good interviewer, and observe this person interacting with your baby, toddler or preschooler often. Your child deserves the best care in all ways every day. You want to leave him or her with someone loving, responsive and knowledgeable – someone your child will look forward to being with every day.

While your child is a baby, seek caregivers who stimulate her language development by talking to her in an animated, but loving way, and respond to her attempts at communication: watching, listening, talking, using exaggerated prosody, responding positively, and making communication joyful. Talk to the caregiver about encouraging speech and language development, and suggest activities listed in the Sharing the Joy sections of this book. Even the most experienced caregivers, who are probably parents themselves, appreciate new ideas for interacting with little ones. Enjoyable, developmentally appropriate activities can bring about great satisfaction as the caregiver watches the baby respond and learn while they both have fun.

If your child is ready for preschool, it is essential to choose a school that employs a well trained staff that will encourage her language growth. Remember that language is the foundation of literacy, and that every day counts. The effect of preschool teachers' professional development in the areas of language and early literacy has been well documented, so the training of the preschool staff will be among the factors included in making your choice. In fact, studies have shown that after well-presented professional development for preschool teachers, even children with somewhat delayed language skills showed marked improvement of language and literacy. Professional development is key.

Visit each preschool you are considering and observe the amount of intellectual challenge the teachers are providing, the frequency of extended conversations children are having with their teachers, and the syntactic complexity of the teachers' language when speaking with the children. Children should be engaged in conversations, expressing and elaborating on their feelings, and commenting on stories read by their teachers. Teachers should be providing feedback to the children's language, asking them open-ended questions, asking follow-up questions and "wh" questions, and quizzing with oral word fill-ins.

Cognitively meaningful talk and experiences help a child understand his world. A combination of planned and guided learning, the opportunity for exploration, and ongoing feedback to the child are all necessary for cognitive development. These experiences can then be integrated into his language repertoire by teachers and parents, and when this happens, he will be motivated to continue to explore and to learn.

Also try this while you are observing at a preschool. See if you can determine whether teachers are thinking about the reasons why having conversations and using book-reading strategies are important. Teachers should not just be using recipes for how to talk and read to children. With real understanding comes flexibility and individualization for each child. Are the teachers changing the complexity of their syntax and vocabulary depending on the children's needs? Some children might need slower, more emphasized speech with directions broken down. Others might need the challenge of more complex sentences and higher-level vocabulary. Are the teachers responding to children's differences?

Do the teachers in this preschool engage children in shared storybook reading in small groups and with individual children? This attention can greatly enhance the development of oral language, vocabulary, comprehension, phonological awareness and print awareness. A lower teacher-to-child ratio while reading and discussing the story allows teachers to really know the needs and potential of each child in order to provide just the right modeling, teaching, and challenges during the reading activity.

As you might expect, kindergarten teachers appreciate children beginning school able to understand and follow directions, demonstrating good social and communication skills, and having a basic knowledge of literacy – book knowledge, writing and beginning spelling. Of course, these skills can be developed by parents, caregivers or preschool teachers. If a lot of your child's time is spent in preschool, though, it needs to be one that prepares him well for kindergarten.

You also need to choose caregivers and preschool teachers who communicate well with parents and who want to work as a cohesive team. Asking each other questions and sharing concerns and observations daily are essential. Have your caregiver write down specific actions and milestones for you that she observes each day, and be clear about what you need and expect. Since infancy and childhood is such important time, you don't want to let a day go by without knowing how your child handled situations, what she said, how she responded to directions – and whether she met any milestones listed in the Stages of Language Developmental chart in Chapter 1: The Basics.

So when deciding upon a preschool that is a good fit for your child, it is wise to ask a number of questions and to observe closely:

➢ What is the **teacher-child ratio** of the preschool? Is there enough staff to give each child the attention he needs? Is there a combination of whole-group teaching/discussion, small group, and individual attention?

➢ Is it a **comforting and welcoming** place? Can you tell that the staff cares for and respects the children? Is there children's art work and dictated stories on the walls? Is there a well-kept play yard that is used daily?

➢ Do the **children seem happy** there? Are they interacting with the staff in a loving and cheerful way?

➢ **Is the staff required to continue to take courses and workshops** in early childhood education, language development, and best practices and strategies for development of the whole child?

➢ Are the teachers and other staff **good models for speech and language**? Do they articulate well, speak slowly and clearly enough for children to understand, use and explain new vocabulary, and use good grammar? Do they at times use some syntax just a little above each child's level in order to teach new sentence structures?

➤ Are the children **working cooperatively**? Are they **sharing** toys and materials? Are they learning social (pragmatic) skills? Do they enjoy being with their classmates?

➤ What is the **philosophy of teaching literacy and math skills**? How is reading and the learning of the alphabet and sounds integrated into each day? Does the staff make the children feel successful with reading and understanding books and stories? Do they read to children, in groups and individually, throughout the day? Are numbers and counting emphasized in daily activities (cooking, taking attendance, distributing snacks, etc.)?

➤ What is **the daily schedule**? Is there a combination of structured activities and ones chosen by each child? Do children have an opportunity to play outside for physical activity every day?

➤ Are there **exploration centers**, like areas for sand and water, art centers, puzzles, dramatic play areas, and block areas? Are their picture books readily available for children to look through?

➤ How does the staff **teach children to resolve conflicts**? Do they emphasize communicating with kind words and listening to each other? What is their approach to teaching social-emotional skills?

➤ **How is discipline handled?** Does the staff involve parents in dealing with behavioral issues? Are appropriate behaviors and rules discussed with the whole class? Are there visual cues that remind children of expected behavior?

➤ **How involved are parents?** Do they volunteer in the classroom? Do they participate in celebrations and special events? How often are parent conferences held?

➤ **Is the preschool accredited** by the state and/or by an organization such as the National Association for the Education of Young Children (NAEYC), the National Association of Independent Schools, or the National Early Childhood Program Accreditation? Have the teachers earned the title of Certified Childcare Professional and/or Child Development Associate?

Author's Ending Thoughts

My hope is that you will use this book as a reference for many years as your child, or children, grow to be proficient communicators and learners. Please share this information with others – friends, family, teachers and caregivers. Since it is organized in a question and answer format, it should be easy for you to pick up and quickly review sections that pertain to your child's current development. Please refer often to the Form-Content-Use Venn diagram of language (Chapter 1). You might bookmark that page. It will remind you of the interaction of all aspects of language so that while you are working on one skill with your child, you can work on other skills at the same time. After a while, this will become second nature to you; you will become your child's best teacher.

Please also visit our web site (www. TheJoyofLanguage. com) often to read *The Joy of Language* blog for additional information and new ideas to try out with your child. There you will also find new research on speech and language development, resources for parents, answers to questions from readers, informal tests and checklists, information about the IEP process at school, case studies, and much more. And please keep in touch. Contact me whenever you have a question or need clarification, or just to say hello. I look forward to being your speech-language consultant, and your friend. Together we can continue to Share the JOY.

My Very Best,

Tara

GLOSSARY OF TERMS

ADD (Attention Deficit Disorder)
A set of behaviors such as impulsivity or lack of focus that can cause learning and behavioral difficulties in school and in social situations. Such symptoms, however, may be caused by factors other than ADD/ADHD, such as intermittent hearing loss, APD or sensory-motor deficits.

ADHD (Attention Deficit Hyperactivity Disorder)
The above characteristics plus hyperactivity.

allophone
A phoneme that sounds slightly different from another but is classified as the same phoneme (e.g., the way /l/ is pronounced at the beginning vs. at the end of a syllable).

APD (Auditory Processing Disorder)
Difficulty for the brain to process auditory information (listening in noisy environments, following directions, discriminating sounds) not caused by hearing loss.

articulation
Movement and placement of the lips, tongue, jaw and teeth for the production of speech.

association
The mental act of pairing concepts with our experiences and current knowledge.

audiogram
Chart that indicates **threshold** hearing (the dB [decibels] and Hz [Hertz or frequency] at which the student is able to detect sound) or **screening** hearing (usually the Hz at which the child hears sound at 25 dB).

auditory discrimination

The ability to discriminate one sound or set of sounds from another.

auditory figure-ground

One's focus on the important auditory information (e.g., the teacher's voice or the voices of others in a cooperative group) without being distracted by other sounds in the environment. Listening to the "figure" vs. the background.

Behavioral Theory

The learning theory that states that a stimulus produces a response, and that response is either rewarded (motivating the responder to repeat the behavior), punished (motivating the responder to avoid the behavior) or extinguished (ending the behavior through ignoring it).

body language

Gestures, postures, and facial expressions that convey meaning.

brain stem

Part of the brain that sits between the spinal cord and the brain and controls basic functions such as breathing, heart rate and blood pressure.

Broca's area

A part of the left hemisphere of the cerebral cortex, discovered by Pierre Paul Broca, that is essential for speech production.

CAPD (see APD)

cerebellum

Located behind the brain stem, it regulates muscle movement, posture, balance and coordination.

child-directed speech (CDS)

The type of sing-songy speech instinctively used to speak to infants and very young children. It was formerly called "motherese."

childhood apraxia of speech (CAS)

A neurological speech disorder which keeps the brain from sending signals to the muscles for correct articulation.

classification

The act of thinking of ideas or concepts as being closely related to each other. Our classification of ideas and concepts changes as we learn more.

coarticulation

The slight changing of a phoneme that occurs as a result of pronouncing previous or subsequent phonemes in an utterance.

cognition

The process of acquiring knowledge and understanding (thinking, regulation of emotional responses, learning and memory).

Cognitive Theory

The learning theory that states that our perceptions, classification of objects and events, and problem solving changes with our experiences (interaction with our environment).

congenital

Inherited by genetic mechanisms. Present at birth.

content

The message, or underlying meaning, of spoken or written language. Semantics.

content words

Those words in an utterance or in written language that carry the meaning: nouns, verbs, adjectives, adverbs and some prepositions.

corpus callosum

The band of nerve fibers between the right and left hemisphere of the brain that is the principal route for communication between the hemispheres.

dB (Decibel)

The intensity (volume) of sound. During a hearing test (audiological exam) dB is charted along the left side of an audiogram.

dialect

Different ways of speaking a language in terms of pronunciation, grammar, vocabulary, idiomatic expressions and social use.

ellipsis

The omission of words from a sentence or conversation that are unnecessary because all participants understand the context.

executive function

Self-management and self-control that includes planning ahead, inhibiting undesirable responses, and holding information in working memory.

form

The phonological, morphological and syntactic systems of spoken and written language.

frontal lobe

The front part (both left and right) of the brain that controls emotions, personality, judgment and speech.

function word

A word in an utterance that functions grammatically, but holds little meaning (articles, conjunctions, prepositions like "of," and auxiliary verbs).

gestalt

Understanding information as it relates to the overall context in which it is used and the context of one's own experiences.

Hz (Hertz)

The cycles per second of the frequency of sound waves that determine the pitch of a sound. Hz is charted along the top of an audiogram.

Innate Theory

A theory of language acquisition that tells us that we, as humans, are born with hypotheses about the rules of language and with the capacity and imperative to learn language.

larynx

The opening in the throat forming the air passage and containing the vocal cords (vocal folds); the "voice box."

language processing

The act of understanding oral and written language when the brain makes appropriate connections for incoming phonemes, morphemes, syntactic structures, vocabulary and social situations.

left hemisphere skills

Receptive and expressive oral and written language skills (phonemic analysis and segmenting, sentence formulation, grammatical rules, formulas) that are processed in the left cerebral hemisphere.

linguistic rules

The myriad of rules that govern word, phrase and sentence formulation.

manner of articulation

The way the breath flows through the mouth resulting in the kind of sound it makes: popping [plosive], friction, nasal, etc.

metacomprehension
The observation and awareness of one's own understanding of oral and written language.

metalinguistic awareness
The awareness that language is an object that can be manipulated, and the understanding of various aspects of language.

morpheme
The smallest unit of meaning of a language. Root words are free morphemes, which can stand alone; morphological inflections are bound morphemes, which only add or change the meaning of a word when they are bound to it. (free = climb; bound = "ed" in climbed)

morphological inflection
A unit of meaning that is added to a root word to change the meaning of the word (prefixes, suffixes, past tense, pluralization, etc.).

motor
Relating to movement.

motor planning
The brain's anticipation of the body motion that is needed to perform tasks – like climbing stairs, writing, or eating with a fork.

neocortex
The newest, or most evolved, portion of the cerebral cortex, involved in higher mental functions.

occipital lobe
The region in the back of the brain that processes visual information.

onset/rime

The initial consonant or consonant cluster (onset) and the vowels and consonants that follow (rime) in a word.

parietal lobe

Located at the top of the brain, behind the frontal lobes. They are responsible for sensations like touch and pressure, spatial relationships, texture, taste, pain, and the internal feeling of our muscles.

phoneme

A sound in a language.

phonemic awareness

The awareness of sounds in spoken words and the awareness of the ability to manipulate those sounds: phoneme isolation, phoneme identity, phoneme categorization, phoneme blending, phoneme segmentation and phoneme deletion.

phonological awareness

The awareness of the sound structure of speech that includes syllables, onset and rime (beginning consonant or consonant cluster and the vowel and consonants that follow) and counting words in a sentence.

place of articulation

The place in the mouth where sound is produced (e.g., between the lips or at the alveolar ridge).

pragmatics

The use of language within the social context. The intent or purpose of the speaker or writer. The intended function of utterances.

prosody

The stresses, intonations and pauses in oral language that carries much of the meaning and intent of the speaker.

right hemisphere skills

Skills of expression and understanding that are based upon tone, rhythm, context/gestalt and visual interpretation. These skills are especially significant for social competence and reading comprehension.

rote memory

The memorization of information or sounds that one does not necessarily understand (e.g., children can memorize the alphabet before they understand its use).

scaffolding

Questioning that leads the learner to discovering the answer to a problem.

semantics

The meaning of spoken and written language, and the way in which we organize and make sense of information.

SMI (Sensory-Motor Integration)

Our brain's ability to organize sensory input (activities, sounds, textures, tastes, images, smells) in order to be able to respond appropriately in a particular situation.

Sensory Processing Disorder (SPD)

An inability to process many types of sensory input at a time (like vision, hearing, balance, and tactile information).

stuttering (also called dysfluency of speech)

The interruption of speech associated with struggle behavior, repetition of sounds or words, overuse of fillers, unusual breathing patterns, facial grimaces, or a number of other behaviors that interrupt the flow of speech.

syntax

The use of grammatical rules to formulate phrases and sentences. It is also referred to as surface structure because the actual meaning of a phrase or sentence cannot always be determined by the sentence structure.

temporal lobe

Located at the bottom middle part of the neocortex, to the sides near the temples. It is responsible for processing (understanding) auditory information (enabling us to make sense of the sounds we hear), other sensory information, and short-term memory.

Theory of Mind

The understanding that other individuals have different knowledge, thoughts and beliefs than ourselves.

vocal cords / vocal folds

Folds of tissue in the larynx that form the glottis, the passage for the airstream that vibrates to produce voice.

voicing

Using the voice (vibration of the vocal cords) to produce phonemes (e.g., /b/, /d/ and /z/).

word retrieval

Also called "word finding." One's ability to recall and use the correct word, a word that the speaker knows, in speaking or writing.

REFERENCES

Aamodt, S. & Wang, S. (2011). *Welcome to your child's brain.* New York: Bloomsbury.

Acredolo, L. & Goodwyn, S. (3rd ed.). (2009). *Baby signs: How to talk with your baby before your baby can talk.* New York: McGraw Hill.

Alanis, I. (2013). Where's your partner? Pairing bilingual learners in preschool and primary grade dual language classrooms. *Young Children 68* (1), 42 – 46.

Altmann, T.R. (ed.). (2006). *The wonder years: Helping your baby and young child successfully negotiate the major developmental milestones.* New York: Bantam Books.

Anderson, A. (1997). Families and mathematics: A study of parent-child interactions. *Journal for Research in Mathematics Education 28* (4), 484 – 511.

Anderson, D., & Pempek, T. (2005). Television and very young children. *The American Behavioral Scientist 48* (5), 505 – 522.

Apel, K. & Lawrence, J. (2011). Contributions to morphological awareness skills to word-level reading and spelling in first-grade children with and without speech sound disorder. *Journal of Speech, Language and Hearing Research 54* (5), 1312 – 1327.

Apel, K. & Masterson, J. (2nd ed.) (2012). *Beyond babytalk.* New York: Three Rivers Press.

Anderson, D., & Pempek, T. (2005). Television and very young children. *American Behavioral Scientist 48*, 505 – 522.

Ashlock, R.B. (1990). Parents can help children learn mathematics. *The Arithmetic Teacher 38* (3), 42 – 46.

Barner, D., Chow, K. & Yang, S. (2009). Finding one's meaning: A test of the relation between quantifiers and integers in language development. *Cognitive Psychology 58*, 195 – 219.

Barnes, B.A. & York, S.M. (2001). *Common sense parenting of toddlers and preschoolers.* Boys Town, NE: Boys Town Press.

Baron, N. (1992). *Growing up with language: How children learn to talk.* Reading, MA: Addison-Wesley.

Barr, R. & Linebarger, D. (2010). Special issue on the content and context of early media exposure. *Infant and Child Development 19* (6), 553 – 556.

Barr, R., Lauricella, A., Zack, E. & Calvert, S. (2010). Infant and early education exposure to adult-directed and child-directed television programming. *Merrill-Palmer Quarterly 56* (1), 21 – 48.

Barry, A. *Linguistic perspectives on language and education.* (2008). Columbus, OH: Pearson.

Beauchat, K., Blamey, K. & Walpole, S. (2009). Building preschool children's language and literacy one storybook at a time. *The Reading Teacher 63* (1), 26 – 39.

Beck, S.W. & Olah, L.N. (eds.) (2001). *Perspectives on language and literacy: Beyond the here and now.* Cambridge, MA: Harvard Educational Review.

Bergelson, E. & Swingley, D. (2012). At 6 – 9 months human infants know the meanings of many common nouns. *Proceedings of the National Academy of Sciences of the United States 109* (9), 3253 – 3258.

Bernard, C. & Gervain, J. (2012). Prosodic cues to word order: What level of representation? *Frontiers in Psychology 3*, 451.

Bittman, M., Rutherford, L., Brown, J. & Unsworth, L. (2012). Digital natives? New and old media and children's language acquisition. *Family Matters 91*, 18.

Bjorklund, C. (2010). Broadening the horizon: Toddlers' strategies for learning mathematics. *International Journal of Early Years Education 18* (1), 71 – 84.

Blachowicz, C. & Obrachta, C. (2005). Vocabulary visits: Virtual field trips for content vocabulary development. *Reading Teacher 59* (3), 262 – 268.

Blanksen, A., O'Brien, M., Leerkes, E., Calkins, S., & Marcovitch, S. (2015). Do hours spent viewing television at ages 3 and 4 predict vocabulary and executive functioning at age 5? *Merrill-Palmer Quarterly 61* (2), 264 – 289.

Blanksen, A., O'Brien, M., Leerkes, E., Marcovitch, S., & Calkins, S. (2011). Shyness and vocabulary: The roles of executive functioning and home environmental stimulation. *Merrill-Palmer Quarterly 57* (2), 105 – 128.

Bloodgood, J.W. (1999). What's in a name? Children's name writing and literacy acquisition. *Teaching Research Quarterly 34* (3), 342 – 367.

Bobb, B. & Casey, B. (2003). The power of block building. *Teaching Children Mathematics 10* (2), 98 – 102.

Bond, M. & Wasik, B. (2009). Conversation stations: Promoting language development in young children. *Early Childhood Education Journal 36* (6), 467 – 473.

Boada, R., Pennington, B., Peterson, R. & Shriberg, L. (2009). What influences literary outcome in children with speech sound disorder? *Journal of Speech, Language and Hearing Research 52* (5), 1175 – 1188.

Brigman, G. & Webb, L. (2003). Ready to learn: Teaching kindergarten students school success skills. *The Journal of Educational Research 96* (5) 286 – 292.

Britto, P.R., Brooks-Gunn, J. & Griffin, T.M. (2006). Maternal reading and teaching patterns: Associations with school readiness in low-income African American families. *Reading Research Quarterly 41* (1), 68 – 89.

Brooks, N., Audet, J. & Barner, D. (2013). Pragmatic inference, not semantic competence, guides 3-year-olds' interpretation of unknown number words. *Developmental Psychology 49* (6), 1066 – 1075.

Bull, R., Espy, K.A. & Wiebe, S. (2008). Short-term memory, working memory and executive functioning in preschoolers: Longitudinal predictors of mathematical achievement at age 7 years. *Developmental Neuropsychology 33* (3), 205 – 228.

Burchinal, M. R., Roberts, J. E., Riggins, R., Jr., Zeisel, S. A., Neebe, E., & Bryant, D. (2000). Relating quality of center-based child care to early cognitive and language development longitudinally. *Child Development 71* (2), 339 – 357.

Butterworth, B. (2005). The development of arithmetical abilities. *Journal of Child Psychology and Psychiatry 46* (1), 3 – 18.

Cain, S. (2012). *Quiet: The power of introverts in a world that can't stop talking.* New York: Broadway Books.

Charlesworth, R. & Leali, S.A. (2011). Using problem solving to assess young children's mathematics knowledge. *Early Childhood Education Journal 39*, 373 – 382.

Cheslock, M.A. & Kahn, S.J. (2011, Sept.20). Supporting families and caregivers in everyday routines. *The ASHA Leader*, 10 – 13.

Christakis, D. (2009). The effects of infant media usage: What do we know and what should we learn? *ACTA Paediatrica 98*, 8 – 16.

Christakis, D., Zimmerman, F., DiGiuseppe, D. & McCarty, C. (2004). Early television exposure and subsequent attentional problems in children. *Pediatrics 113* (4), 708 – 713.

Clark, C.A.C., Sheffield, T.D., Wiebe, S.A. & Espy, K.A. (2013). Longitudinal associations between executive control and developing mathematical competence in preschool boys and girls. *Child Development 84* (2), 662 – 677.

Clements, D.H. (1999). Subitizing: What is it? Why teach it? *Teaching Children Mathematics 5* (7), 400 – 405.

Clements, D.H. (2003). Math: A civil right. *Early Childhood Today 17* (4), 4.

Clements, D.H. & Sarama, J. (2004). Mathematics everywhere, every time. *Teaching Children Mathematics 10* (8), 421 – 426.

Coleman, C. (2013, Sept. 26). How can you tell if childhood stuttering is the real deal? *ASHAsphere*. Retrieved June 23, 2014, from http://blog.asha.org/?s=stuttering

Collins, M.F. (2010). ELL Preschoolers' english vocabulary acquisition from storybook reading. *Early Childhood Research Quarterly 25* (1), 84 – 97.

Colonnesi, C., Stams, G.J.J.M., Koster, I., & Noom, M.J. (2010). The relation between pointing and language development: A meta-analysis. *Developmental Review 30* (4), 352 – 66.

Chonchaiya, W. & Pruksananonda, C. (2008). Television viewing associates with delayed language development. *Acta Paediatrica 97* (7), 977 – 982.

Condry, K.F. & Spelke, E.S. (2008). The development of language and abstract concepts: The case of natural number. *Journal of Experimental Psychology: General 137* (1), 22 – 38.

Connor, C., Morrison, F. & Slominski, L. (2006). Preschool instruction and children's emergent literacy growth. *Journal of Educational Psychology 98* (4), 665 – 689.

Cooper, S. (2010). Lighting up the brain with songs and stories. *General Music Today 23* (2), 24 – 30.

Courage, M. & Howe, M. (2010). To watch or not to watch: Infants and toddlers in a brave new electronic world. *Developmental Review 30* (2), 101 – 115.

Cox, R., Skouteris, H., Dell'Aquila, D., Hardy, L., & Rutherford, L. (2013). Television viewing behavior among preschoolers: Implications for public health recommendations. *Journal of Pediatrics & Child Health 49* (2), 108 – 111.

Cuperus, J., Hermans, S., Jansonius, K., Ketelaars, M. & Verhoeven, L. (2011). Semantic abilities of children with pragmatic language impairment: The case of picture naming skills. *Journal of Speech, Language and Hearing Research 54* (1), 87 – 98.

Craig-Unkefer, L., & Kaiser, A. (2002). Improving the social communication of at-risk preschool children in a play context. *Topics in Early Childhood Special Education 22* (1), 3 – 13.

Dauksas, L. & White, J. (2014). Discovering shapes and space in preschool. *Teaching Young Children 7* (4), 22 – 25.

Deckner, D.F., Adamson, L.B. & Bakeman, R. (2006). Child and maternal contributions to shared reading: Effects on language and literacy development. *Journal of Applied Developmental Psychology 27* (1), 31 – 41.

DeLoache, J.S. & Korac, N. (2003). Video based learning by very young children. *Developmental Science 6* (3), 245 – 246.

DeLoache, J.S., Chiong, C., Sherman, K., Islam, N., Vanderborght, M., Troseth, G., Strouse, G.A. & O'Doherty, K. (2010). Do babies learn from baby media? *Psychological Science 21* (11), 1570 – 1574.

DeLuzio, J. & Girolametto, L. (2011). Peer interactions of preschool children with and without hearing loss. *Journal of Speech, Language and Hearing Research 54* (4), 1197 – 1210.

Denham, S., Blair, K., DeMulder, E., Levitas, J., Sawyer, K., Auerbach-Major, S. & Queenan, P. (2003). Preschool emotional competence: Pathway to social competence? *Child Development 74* (1), 238 – 256.

Desoete, A. & Gregoire, J. (2006). Numerical competence in young children and in children with mathematics learning disabilities. *Learning and Individual Differences 16* (4), 351 – 367.

Dickenson, D. & Caswell, L. (2007). Building support for language and early literacy in preschool classrooms through in-service professional development: Effects of the literacy environment enrichment program. *Early Childhood Research Quarterly 22* (2), 243 – 260.

Dickinson, D., McCabe, A., Anastasopoulos, L., Peisner-Feinberg, E., & Poe, M. (2003). The comprehensive language approach to early literacy: The interrelationships among vocabulary, phonological sensitivity, and print knowledge among preschool-aged children. *Journal of Educational Psychology 95*, (3), 465 – 481.

Dickinson, D. K., & Tabors, P. O. (eds.). (2001). *Beginning literacy with language: Young children learning at home and school.* Baltimore, MD: Brookes Publishing.

Drake, K., Belsky, J. and Pasco Fearon, R.M. (2014). From early attachment to engagement with learning in school: The role of self-regulation and persistence. *Developmental Psychology 50* (5), 1350 – 1361.

Duncan, G.J, Dowsett, C.J., Claessens, A., Magnuson, K., Huston, A.C., Klebanov, P., Pagani, L.S., … Japel, C. (2007). School readiness and later achievement. *Developmental Psychology 43* (6), 1428 – 1446.

Dunckley, V. (2015). *Reset your child's brain: A four-week plan to end meltdowns, raise grades and boost social skills by reversing the effects of electronic screen time.* Novato, CA: New World Library.

Edens, K.M. & Potter, E.F. (2012). An exploratory look at the relationships among math skills, motivational factors and activity choice. *Early Childhood Education Journal 41*, 235 – 243.

Estes, K.G. & Bowen, S. (2013). Learning about sounds contributes to learning about words: effects of prosody and phonotactics on infant word learning. *Journal of Experimental Psychology 114* (3), 405 – 417.

Farrant, B. (2012). Joint attention and parent-child book reading: Keys to help close gaps in early language development, school readiness and academic achievement. *Family Matters 91*, 38 – 46.

Fender, J., Richert, R., Robb, M., & Wartella, E. (2010). Parent teaching focus and toddlers' learning from an infant DVD. *Infant and Child Development 19* (6), 613 – 627.

Fenstermacher, S., Barr, R., Brey, E., Pempek, T., Ryan, M., Calvert, S., Shwery, C., & Linebarger, D. (2010). Interactional quality depicted in infant and toddler videos: Where are the interactions? *Infant and Child Development 19*, 594 – 612.

Ferguson, C. & Donnellen, M. (2014). Is the association between children's baby video viewing and poor language development robust? A reanalysis of Zimmerman, Christakis and Meltzoff (2007). *Developmental Psychology 50* (1), 129 – 137.

Ferguson, M.A., Hall, R.L., Riley, A. & Moore, D.R. (Feb., 2011). Communication, listening, cognitive and speech perception skills in children with auditory processing disorder (APD) or specific language impairment (SLI). *Journal of Speech, Language and Hearing Research 54*, 211 – 227.

Fidler, A., Zack, E., & Barr, R. (2010). Television viewing patterns in 6- to 18-month-olds: The role of caregiver-infant interactional quality. *Infancy 15* (2), 176 – 196.

Flynn, K.S. (2011, Nov./Dec.). Developing children's oral language skills through dialogic reading: Guidelines for implementation. *Teaching Exceptional Children*, 8 – 16.

Fox, J. & Lee, J. (2009). Children's communication and socialization skills by types of early education experience. *Journal of Research in Childhood Education 23* (4), 475 – 488.

Freeman, David E. & Yvonne F. Freeman (2004). *Essential linguistics: What you need to know to teach reading, ESL, spelling, phonics, grammar.* Heinemann: Portsmouth, NH.

Geist, K. & Geist, E.A. (2008). Do re mi, 1 – 2 – 3: That's how easy math can be: Using music to support emerging mathematics. *Young Children 63* (2), 20 – 25.

Genesee, F. (2009). Early childhood bilingualism: Perils and possibilities. *Journal of Applied Research in Learning 2 (Special Issue)* (2), 1 – 21.

Gentile, D., Oberg, C., Sherwood, N., Story, M., Walsh, D. & Hogan, M. (2004). Well-child visits in the video age: Pediatricians and the American academy of pediatrics' guidelines for children's media use. *Pediatrics 114* (5), 1235 – 1241.

Gervain, J., Berent, I. & Werker, J. (2012). Binding at birth: The newborn brain detects identity relations and sequential position in speech. *Journal of Cognitive Neuroscience 24* (3), 564 – 574.

Gillanders, C. (2007). An English-speaking prekindergarten teacher for young Latino children: Implications of the teacher-child relationship on second language learning. *Early Childhood Education Journal 35*, (1), 47 – 54.

Gillon, G. (2002). Phonological awareness intervention for children. *ASHA Leader 7* (22), 4 – 17.

Goldenberg, C., Hicks, J. & Lit, I. (2013). Dual language learners: Effective instruction in early childhood. *American Educator 37* (2), 26 – 29.

Golinkoff, R. & Hirsh-Pasek, K. (2006). Baby wordsmith. *Current Directions in Psychological Science 15* (1), 30 – 33.

Golinkoff, R. & Hirsh-Pasek, K. (2000). *How babies talk: The magic and mystery of language in the first three years of life.* New York: Penguin Group.

Goodwin, B. (2012, March). Address reading problems early. *Educational Leadership,* 80 – 81.

Gratier, M., & Devouche, E. (2011). Imitation and repetition of prosodic contour in vocal interaction at 3 months. *Developmental Psychology 47* (1), 67 – 76.

Greenes, C., Ginsburg, H.P. & Balfanz, R. (2004). Big math for little kids. *Early Childhood Research Quarterly 19* (1), 159 – 166.

Grigos, M. & Patel, R. (2007). Articulator movement associated with the development of prosodic control in children. *Journal of Speech, Language and Hearing Research 50* (1), 119 – 130.

Guglielmo, H.M. (2001). Social skill training in an integrated preschool program. *School Psychology Quarterly 16* (2), 158 – 175.

Gulay, H. (2011). The evaluation of the relationship between the TV-viewing habits and peer relations of preschool children. *International Journal of Academic Research 3* (2), 922 – 930.

Guven, Y. (2009). The factors related to preschool children and their mothers on children's intuitional mathematics abilities. *International Journal of Science and Mathematics Education 7* (3), 533 – 549.

Halsey, C. (2012) *Baby development: Everything you need to know.* New York: Dorling Kindersley Limited.

Hamer, M., Stamatakis, E. & Mishra, G. (2009). Psychological distress, television viewing and physical activity in children aged 4 to 12 years. *Pediatrics 123* (5), 1263 – 1268.

Hart, B. & Risley, T.R. (2003). The early catastrophe: The 30-million word gap by age 3. *American Educator 27* (1), 4 – 9.

Henrichs, J., Rescorla, L., Donkersloot, C., Schenk, J., Raat H. & Jaddoe V. (2013). Early vocabulary delay and behavioral/emotional problems in early childhood: The generation R study. *Journal of Speech, Language and Hearing Research 56* (2), 553 – 566.

Hepach, R., Vaish, A. & Tomasello, M. (2013). Young children sympathize less in response to unjustified emotional distress. *Developmental Psychology 49* (6), 1132 – 1138.

Herold, D., Nygaard, L., & Namy, L. (2012). Say it like you mean it: mothers' use of prosody to convey word meaning. *Language and Speech 55* (3), 423 – 436.

Hinitz, B.S.F. (2014, May). Head Start: A bridge from past to future. *Young Children*. (National Association for the Education of Young Children), 94 – 97.

Hoff, E. (2003). The specificity of environmental influence: Socioeconomic status affects early vocabulary development via maternal speech. *Child Development 74* (5), 1368 – 1378.

Holland, J. (2008). Reading aloud with infants: The controversy, the myth and a case study. *Early Childhood Education Journal 35* (4), 383 – 385.

Holmes, A. & Huston, E. (2010). Understanding positive father-child interaction: Children's, fathers', and mothers' contributions. *Fathering 8* (2), 203 – 225.

Howes, C. (1997). Children's experiences in center-based child care as a function of teacher background and adult–child ratio. *Merrill-Palmer Quarterly, 43* (3), 404 – 425.

Jentschke, S., Koelsch, S., Sallat, S. & Friederici, A. (2008). Children with specific language impairment also show impairment of music-syntactic processing. *Journal of Cognitive Neuroscience 20* (11), 1940 – 1951.

Jacobson, L. (2001). Early Years. *Education Week 20* (38), 9.

Jalongo, M. & Sobolak, M. (2011). Supporting young children's vocabulary growth: The challenges, benefits, and evidence-based strategies. *Early Childhood Education Journal 38* (6), 24 – 29.

Kamuran, T. (2009). The effects of cooperative learning on preschoolers' mathematics problem-solving ability. *Educational Studies in Mathematics 72* (3), 325 – 340.

Kindle, K. (2009). Vocabulary development during read-alouds: Primary practices. *The Reading Teacher 63* (3), 202 – 211.

Kirkorian, H., Pempek, T., Murphy, L., Schmidt, M. and Anderson, D. (2009). The impact of background television on parent-child interaction. *Child Development 80* (5), 1350 – 1359.

Klibanoff, R.S., Levine, S.C., Huttenlocher, J., Vasilyeva, M. & Hedges, L.V. (2006). Preschool children's mathematical knowledge: The effect of teacher "math talk." *Developmental Psychology 42* (1), 59 – 69.

Kovács, A.M. & Mehler, J. (2009). Cognitive gains in 7-month old bilingual infants. *Proceedings of the National Academy of Sciences 106* (16), 6556 – 6560.

Krajewski, K. & Schneider, W. (2009). Exploring the impact of phonological awareness, visual-spatial working memory, and preschool quantity-number competencies on mathematics achievement in elementary school: Findings from a 3-year longitudinal study. *Journal of Experimental Child Psychology 103* (4), 516 – 531.

Krcmar, M., Grela, B. & Lin, K. (2007). Can toddlers learn vocabulary from television? An experimental approach. *Median Psychology 10*, 41 – 63.

Krieger, L. (2013). The effects of improvisational music therapy on joint attention behaviors in autistic children: A randomized controlled study. *Journal of Autism & Developmental Disorders 38* (9), 1758 – 1766.

Lally, J.R. & Mangione, P. (2013). Building infant and toddler intellect and language on a social-emotional base: The developmentally appropriate roots of school readiness. (Presentation at NAEYC's 2010 *National Institute for Early Childhood Professional Development*).

Lapierre, M., Piotrowski, J. & Linebarger, D. (2012). Background television in the homes of U.S. children. *Pediatrics 130* (5), 839 – 846.

Lawson, K. (2012). The real power of parental reading aloud: Exploring the affective and attentional dimensions. *Australian Journal of Education 56* (3), 257 – 272.

Lee, J.S. and Ginsburg, H.P. (2009). Early childhood teachers' misconceptions about mathematics education for young children in the United States. *Australasian Journal of Early Childhood 34* (4), 37 – 45.

Lefevre, J., Fast, L., Skwarchuk, S., Smith-Chant, B.L., Bisanz, J., Kamawar, D. & Penner-Wilger, M. (2010). Pathways to mathematics: Longitudinal predictors of performance. *Child Development 81* (6), 1753 – 1767.

Leung, C. (2008). Preschoolers' acquisition of scientific vocabulary through repeated read-aloud events, retellings and hands-on science activities. *Reading Psychology 29* (2), 165 – 193.

Lillard, A. & Peterson, J. (2011). The immediate impact of different types of television on young children's executive function. *Pediatrics 128* (4), 644 – 649.

Linebarger, D. & Walker, D. (2005). Infants' and toddlers' television viewing and language outcomes. *The American Behavioral Scientist 48* (5), 624 – 645.

Linebarger, D. & Piotrowski, J. (2009). TV as storyteller: How exposure to television impacts at-risk preschoolers' story knowledge and narrative skills. *British Journal of Developmental Psychology 27* (1), 47 – 69.

Lipsey, M.W., Farran, D.C. & Hofer, K.G. (2015). A randomized control trial of a statewide voluntary prekindergarten program of children's skills and behaviors through third grade. *Peabody Research Institute.* Vanderbilt University, Nashville, TN.

Lipton, J.S. & Spelke, E.S. (2006). Preschool children master the logic of number word meanings. *Cognition 98* (3), B57 – B66.

Mackesey, T. (2013). Early intervention for stuttering: A time for grassroots advocacy. *The ASHA Leader 18* (10), 4

Manfra, L., Dinehart, L. H. B. & Sembiante, S.F. (2014). Associations between counting ability in preschool and mathematic performance in first grade among a sample of ethnically diverse, low income children. *Journal of Research in Childhood Education 28* (1), 101 – 114.

Mayes, L.C. & Cohen, D.J. (2002) *The Yale Child Study Center guide to understanding your child.* New York: Little Brown and Co.

Maxim, G.W. (1989). Developing preschool mathematical concepts. *The Arithmetic Teacher 37* (4), 36 – 41.

McCrea, E. (2014) The power of early identification. *The ASHA Leader 19* (2), 8 – 9.

Merriam-Webster.com. 2016. http://www.merriam-webster.com

Moomaw, S. & Davis, J.A. (2010). STEM comes to preschool. *Young Children 65* (5), 12 – 14, 16 – 18.

Moore, D.R. (2007). Auditory processing disorders: Acquisition and Treatment. *Journal of Communication Disorders 40* (4), 295 – 304.

Mumme, D. L., & Fernald, A. (2003). The infant as on-looker: Learning from emotional reactions observed in a television scenario. *Child Development 74* (1), 221 – 237.

Mulsow, M. & Stevens, T. (2006). There is no meaningful relationship between television exposure and symptoms of attention-deficit/hyperactivity disorder. *Pediatrics 117* (4), 665 – 672.

Napier, C. (2014). How use of screen and media affects the emotional development of infants. *Primary Health Care 24* (2), 18 – 25.

Nathanson, A. & Rasmussen, E. (2011). TV viewing compared to book reading and toy playing reduces responsive maternal communication with toddlers and preschoolers. *Human Communication Research 37*, 465 – 487.

Nathanson, A., Sharp, M., Alade, F., Rasmussen, E. & Christy, K. (2013). The relation between television exposure and Theory of Mind among preschoolers. *Journal of Communication 63*, 1088 – 1108.

National Institute of Child Health and Human Development, Early Child Care Research Network. (2009). Family-peer linkages: The mediational role of attentional processes. *Social Development 18* (4), 875 – 895.

Negen, J. & Sarnecka, B. (2012). Number-concept acquisition and general vocabulary development. *Child Development 83* (6), 2019 – 2027.

Neu, R.A. (2013). An exploration of oral language development in Spanish-speaking preschool students. *Early Childhood Education Journal 41*(3), 211 – 218.

Neuman, S.B. (2014). Content-rich instruction in preschool. *Educational Leadership 72* (2), 36 – 40.

Neuman, S. B., & Dickinson, D. K. (2001). *Handbook of early literacy research.* New York, NY: Guilford Press.

Neuman, S. B., Kaefer, T., Pinkham, A., & Strouse, G. (2014). Can babies learn to read? A randomized trial of baby media. *Journal of Educational Psychology 106* (3), 815 – 830.

NICHD ECCRN. (2000). The relation of child care to cognitive and language development. *Child Development 71* (4), 960 – 980.

Nielsen, D., Friesen, L. & Fink, J. (2011 – 2012). The effectiveness of a model of language-focused classroom instruction on the vocabulary and narrative development of kindergarten children. *Journal of Education 92* (2), 63 – 77.

Nunes, T. & Bryant, P. (2004). Morphological awareness. *Literacy Today 38*, 18 – 19.

Nys, J., Content, A. & Leybaert, J. (2013). Impact of language abilities on exact and approximate number skills development: Evidence from children with specific language impairment. *Journal of Speech, Language and Hearing Research 56* (3) 956 – 970.

Passolunghi, M.C., Vercelloni, B. & Schadee, H. (2007). The precursors of mathematics learning: Working memory, phonological ability and numerical competence. *Cognitive Development 22* (2), 165 – 184.

Páez, M. & Rinaldi, C. (2006). Predicting English word reading skills for Spanish-speaking students in first grade. *Topics in Language Disorders 26* (4), 338 – 350.

Pempek, T., Kirkorian, H., Richards, J., Anderson, D., Lund, A. & Stevens, M. (2010). Video comprehensibility and attention in very young children. *Developmental Psychology 46* (5), 1283 – 1293.

Petersen, I., Bates, J., D'Onofrio, B., Coyne, C., Lansford, J., Dodge, K., Pettit G. & Van Hulle, C. (2013). Language ability predicts the development of behavior problems in children. *Journal of Abnormal Psychology 122* (2), 542 – 557.

Phillips, D., Mekos, D., Scarr, S., McCartney, K., & Abbott Shim, M. (2001). Within and beyond the classroom door: Assessing quality in child care centers. *Early Childhood Research Quarterly 15* (4), 475 – 496.

Piker, R.A. (2013). Understanding influences of play on second language learning: A microethnographic view in one Head Start preschool classroom. *Journal of Early Childhood Research 11* (2), 184 – 200.

Purpura, D.J. and Lonigan, C.J. (2013). Informal numeracy skills: The structure and relations among numbering, relations and arithmetic operations in preschool. *American Educational Research Journal 50* (1), 178 – 209.

Richard, G.J. (July, 2011). The role of the speech-language pathologist in identifying and treating children with auditory processing disorder. *Language, Speech and Hearing Services in Schools 42*, 241 – 245.

Robb, M., Richert, R., & Wartella, E. (2009). Just a talking book? Word learning from watching baby videos. *British Journal of Developmental Psychology 27* (1), 27– 45.

Roggman, L., Boyce, L., Cook, G., Christiansen, K. & Jones, D. (2004). Playing with daddy: Social toy play, early Head Start, and developmental outcomes. *Fathering 2* (1), 83 – 108.

Rowe, M., Raudenbush, S. & Goldin-Meadow, S. (2012). The pace of vocabulary growth helps predict later vocabulary skill. *Child Development 83* (2), 508 – 525.

Ruston, H.P. & Schwanenflugel, P.J. (2010). Effects of a conversation intervention on the expressive vocabulary development of prekindergarten children. *Language, Speech & Hearing Services in the Schools 43* (3), 303 – 313.

Ryan, A. & Logue-Kennedy, M. (2013). Exploration of teachers' awareness and knowledge of (Central) Auditory Processing Disorder ((C)APD). *British Journal of Special Education 40* (4), 167 – 174.

Sarama, J. & Clements, D.H. (2003). Building blocks of early childhood mathematics. *Teaching Children Mathematics 9* (8), 480 – 484.

Sarnecka, B.W. & Carey, S. (2008). How counting represents number: What children must learn and when they learn it. *Cognition 108* (3), 662 – 674.

Sarnecka, B.W. & Gelman, S.A. (2004). Six does not just mean a lot: Preschoolers see number words as specific. *Cognition 92* (3), 329 – 352.

Schickendanz, J.A. & Collins, M.F. (2013). *So much more than the ABCs: The early phases of reading and writing.* Washington, DC: National Association for the Education of Young Children.

Schmidt, M.E., Pempek, T.A., Kirkorian, H.L., (2008). The effects of background television on toy play behavior of very young children. *Child Development 79* (4), 1137 – 1151.

Schmidt, M. & Vandewater, E. (2008). Media and attention, cognition and school achievement. *The Future of Children 18* (1), 63 – 85.

Seidl, A., Tincoff, R., Baker, C. & Cristia, A. (2014). Why the body comes first: Effects of experimenter touch on infants' word finding. *Developmental Science.* doi: 10.1111/desc.12182

Senechal, M. & LeFevre, J. (2002). Parental involvement in the development of children's reading skill. *Child Development 73* (2), 445 – 460.

Shaywitz, S. (2003). *Overcoming dyslexia: A new and complete science-based program for reading problems at any level.* New York: Alfred A. Knopf.

Shiakalli, M.A. & Zacharos, K. (2012). The contribution of external representations in pre-school mathematical problem solving. *International Journal of Early Years Education 20* (4), 315 – 331.

Singh, L., Reznick, J.S., & Xuehua, L. (2012). Infant word segmentation and childhood vocabulary development: A longitudinal analysis. *Developmental Science 15* (4), 482 – 495.

Smith, V., Mirenda, P. & Zaidman-Zait, A. (2007). Predictors of expressive vocabulary growth in children with autism. *Journal of Speech, Language and Hearing Research 50* (1), 149 – 160.

Sophian, C. (2002). Learning about what fits: Preschool children's reasoning about effects of object size. *Journal for Research in Mathematics Education 33* (4), 290 – 302.

Smit, A.B, Hand, L., Freilinger, J.J., Bernthal, J.E. & Bird, A. (1990). The Iowa articulation norms project and its Nebraska replication. *Journal of Speech and Hearing Disorders, 55*, 779 – 798.

Starkey, P., Klein, A. and Wakeley, A. (2004). Enhancing young children's mathematical knowledge through a pre-kindergarten mathematics intervention. *Early Childhood Research Quarterly 19* (1), 99 – 120.

Stiles, J. & Stern, C. (2001). Developmental change in spatial cognitive processing: Complexity effects and block construction performance in preschool children. *Journal of Cognition and Development 2* (2), 157 – 187.

Sticht, T.G. (2012). Getting it right from the start: The case for early parenthood education. *Education Digest 77* (9), 11 – 17.

Stockall, N. (2011). Cooperative groups: Engaging elementary students with pragmatic language impairments. *Teaching Exceptional Children 44* (2), 18 – 25.

Storkel, H., Maekawa, J. & Aschenbrenner, A. (2013). The effect of homonymy on learning correctly articulated vs. misarticulated words. *Journal of Speech, Hearing and Language Research 56* (2), 694 – 707.

Strauss, V. (September 30, 2015). Why parents should talk a lot to their young kids – and choose their words carefully. *The Washington Post.* Retrieved from https://www.washingtonpost.com/news/answer-sheet/wp/2015/09/30/why-parents-should-talk-a-lot-to-their-young-kids-and-choose-their-words-carefully/

Suskind, D. (2015). *Thirty million words: Building a child's brain.* New York, NY: Dutton.

Swingley, D. (2008). The roots of early vocabulary in infants' learning from speech. *Current Directions in Psychological Science 17* (5), 308 – 312.

Tamis-LeMonda, C.S., Shannon, J .D., Cabrera, N.J., & Lamb, M.E. (2004). Fathers and mothers at play with their 2- and 3-year-olds: Contributions to language and cognitive development. *Child Development 75* (6), 1806 – 1820.

Thakkar, R., Garrison, M. & Christakis, D. (2006). A systematic review for the effects of television viewing by infants and preschoolers. *Pediatrics 118* (5), 2025 – 2031.

Thomas, J. (2012). Language play for infants: Man in the moon for male caregivers. *Australasian Public Libraries and Information Services 25* (2), 71 – 75.

Thompson, D. & Christakis, D. (2005). The association between television viewing and irregular sleep schedules among children less than 3 years of age. *Pediatrics 16* (4), 851 – 856.

Toddler development hurt by TV viewing, study finds. (September, 2005). *The Brown University Child and Adolescent Behavior Letter, 7.*

Troseth, G., Saylor, M. & Archer, A. (2006). Young children's use of video as a source of socially relevant information. *Child Development 77* (3), 786 – 799.

University of Hertfordshire. (2012, October 4). Signing in babies does not accelerate language development, study suggests. *Science Daily.* Retrieved February 2, 2015 from www.sciencedaily.com/releases/2012/10/121004093155.htm

University of Washington. (2014, July 14). Months before their first words, babies' brains rehearse speech mechanics. *Science Daily.* Retrieved February 2, 2015 from www.sciencedaily.com/releases/2014/07/140714152311.htm

U.S. Department of Education. (2013, February). *What Works Clearinghouse: Social Skills Training.* Retrieved March 12, 2014 from http://ies.ed.gov/ncee/wwc/pdf/intervention_reports/wwc_socialskills_020513.pdf

Vaala, S., Linebarger, D., Fenstermacher, S., Tedone, A., Brey, E., Barr, R., Moses, A., Shwery, C. & Calvert, S. (2010). Content analysis of language-promoting teaching strategies in infant-directed media. *Infant and Child Development 19*, 628 – 648.

Vaala, S. & LaPierre, M. (2014). Marketing genius: The impact of educational claims and cues on parents' reactions to infant/toddler DVDs. *The Journal of Consumer Affairs 48* (2), 323 – 350.

Verdine, B.N., Irwin, C.M., Golinkoff, R.M. & Hirsh-Pasek, K. (2014, October). Contributions of executive function and spatial skills to preschool mathematics achievement. *Journal of Experimental Child Psychology 126*, 37 – 51.

Verhoeven, L. & Van Leeuwe, J. (2008). Prediction of the development of reading comprehension. *Applied Cognitive Psychology 22* (3), 407 – 423.

Waldman, D. & Roush, J. (2005). *Your Child's Hearing Loss: What Parents Need to Know.* New York: Penguin Group.

Wasik, B. & Hindman, A. (2011). Improving vocabulary and pre-literacy skills of at-risk preschoolers through teacher professional development. *Journal of Educational Psychology 103* (2), 455 – 469.

Wasik, B., Bond, M. & Hindman, A. (2006). The effects of language and literacy intervention on Head Start children and teachers. *Journal of Educational Psychology 98* (1), 63 – 74.

Webster, L., Low, J., Siller, C. & Hackett, R. (2013), Understanding the importance of father's warmth on his child's social skills. *Fathering 11* (1), 90 – 113.

White-Schwoch, T., Woodruff Carr, K., Thompson, E.C., Anderson, S., Nicol, T., et al. (2015). Auditory processing in noise: A preschool biomarker for literacy. *PLoS Biology 13* (7).

Williams, B.H. (2011, April 5). Enhancing phonological patterns of young children with highly unintelligible speech. *The ASHA Leader*, 16 – 19.

Willinger, U. & Eisenwort, B. (2005). Mothers' estimates of their children with disorders of language development. *Behavioral Medicine 31* (3), 117 – 124.

Woolfson, R.C. (2002) *Small talk*. Hauppauge, NY: Barron's.

Yoshinaga-Itano, C. (2011, September 20). Achieving optimal outcomes from EHDI. *The ASHA Leader*, 14 – 17.

Zampini, L. & D'Odorico, L. (2009). Communicative gestures and vocabulary development in 36-month old children with Down's syndrome. *International Journal of Language and Communication Disorders 44* (6) 1063 – 1073.

INDEX